Lecture Notes in Biomathematics

Managing Editor: S. Levin

75

Helmut Knolle

Cell Kinetic Modelling and the Chemotherapy of Cancer

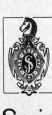

Springer-Verlag

Berlin Heidelberg New York London Paris Tokyo

Author

Helmut Knolle
Medizinische Hochschule Hannover
Abteilung für Epidemiologie und Sozialmedizin
Postfach 61 180, 3000 Hannover 61, Federal Republic of Germany

Mathematics Subject Classification (1980): 34-04, 34 E 99, 92 A 07

ISBN 3-540-50153-3 Springer-Verlag Berlin Heidelberg New York
ISBN 0-387-50153-3 Springer-Verlag New York Berlin Heidelberg

PREFACE

During the last 30 years, many chemical compounds that are active against tumors have been discovered or developed. At the same time, new methods of testing drugs for cancer therapy have evolved. Before 1964, drug testing on animal tumors was directed to observation of the increase in life span of the host after a single dose. A new approach, in which the effects of multiple doses on the proliferation kinetics of the tumor in vivo as well as of cell lines in vitro are investigated, has been outlined by Skipper and his co-workers in a series of papers beginning in 1964 (Skipper, Schabel and Wilcox, 1964 and 1965). They also investigated the influence of the time schedule in the treatment of experimental tumors. Since the publication of those studies, cell population kinetics cannot be left out of any discussion of the rational basis of chemotherapy.

When clinical oncologists began to apply cell kinetic concepts in practice about 15 years ago, the theoretical basis was still very poor, in spite of Skipper's progress, and the lack of re-levant cytokinetic and pharmacologic data was apparent. Subsequently, much theoretical work has been done and many cell kinetic models have been elaborated (for a review see Eisen, 1977). The number of papers dealing with mathematical modelling of chemotherapy is surprising, but the application of mathematical methods to the design of treatment protocols is still hampered by severe problems, one of which is the lack of data describing the action of the drugs used in cancer therapy. The thesis of this monograph is that the next step towards 'mathematical chemotherapy' should be the design of methods suited to determining the action parameters of cytotoxic drugs.

This task cannot be approached without some insight into the growth kinetics of unperturbed cell populations. Therefore, Chapter I of this book presents the basic facts of cell proliferation and some mathematical models of population growth. The first two sections are written for the mathematician who is beginning to work in the area. In Chapter II the mathematical evaluation of some cell kinetic experiments without drug effects is treated in a systematic fashion; this may be useful for the experimental research worker who needs a mathematical guide in the design and evaluation of his experiments. The reader who is interested in the analysis of DNA-histograms from flow cytophotometry is referred to other texts (Eisen 1977, Zietz and Nicolini 1978). In Chapter III various effects of cytotoxic agents are described in mathematical terms, experiments for the measurement of action parameters are discussed and their evaluation analysed. Finally, computer simulations of the action of cytotoxic drugs on cell populations are presented.

All the models in Chapter I are simplified images of reality, in that they are represented by linear equations (having exponential solutions) and neglect the spatial structure of

tissues and solid tumors. Now it is known that the growth of
most tumors at the clinical stage is not exponential, due to
increasing cell loss or changes of other cell kinetic
parameters. But if we intend to study the behavior of cell
populations within a range of a few days or weeks during which
several doses of drugs are administered, then those long term
changes of parameters may be neglected and linear equations are
a good approximation. Furthermore, chemotherapy is often applied
after disappearance of detectable tumor burdens and in the
prevention of metastases, where exponential tumor growth is
rather probable. Among many possible linear models, I have
selected that of Takahashi. This is because, at least in the
field of leukemia where chemotherapy is most frequently used, it
admits a sufficient degree of complexity without unreasonably
increasing the computational effort.

These notes are intended to be a guide to mathematical cell
kinetics for oncologists, and also to enable mathematicians to
acquire the background needed to discuss and collaborate with
medical and biological researchers. Therefore, I have tried to
attain a level of mathematical rigor and complexity midway
between the experimentally oriented booklet by Aherne,
Camplejohn and Wright (1977) and the highly involved
presentation of cell kinetics in the last chapter of the
monograph on branching processes by Jagers (1975). Consequently,
more complex models that include e.g. the correlation between
cycle times of mother and daughter cells are not considered. On
the other hand, a version of the Takahashi model with periodic
coefficients is treated thoroughly in the Appendix and plays an

important role in the simulation studies of chemotherapy described in Chapter III.

The author is grateful to Brigitte Maurer-Schultze, Joannis Bassukas and Gerd Hagemann for helpful comments on Chapter II and III, and to Ilka Lee and Simon Levin for their editorial work. I am also indebted to Gerhard Nehmiz for assistance in computer programming, to Colin Davies for help in translating, to Sabine Siegismund for illustration and to Hildegard Schmeetz for assistance in typing. The final manuscript was expertly typed by Thomas Dahle. Financial support from the Federal Ministry of Research and Technology is gratefully acknowledged.

Hannover, January 1987

Helmut Knolle

CONTENTS

Chapter III . Cell kinetics and cancer therapy

Appendix

I. MATHEMATICAL MODELS OF CELL POPULATIONS

1. Proliferation and differentiation of cells

Reproduction or proliferation is the most characteristic feature of
life. Higher living organisms are composed of millions of cells, which
are organized into tissues and organs. But only cells, those atoms of
life, and organisms are endowed with the capacity of proliferation.
It is inconceivable that a liver could produce a second liver, but
the liver cells are capable of proliferating and therefore the liver
can regenerate itself after partial resection, a fact already told
by Greek mythology.

In nature there is a variety of different modes of reproduction. Cells
reproduce themselves by division. In animals, sexual reproduction pre-
vails. Although the modes of reproduction are qualitatively distinct,
the quantitative description of the population kinetics can often be
achieved by the same mathematical model. The one-sex model of population biology, which considers only females, is suited for cell populations as well as for animal populations with abundance of males.
This fact is reflected very well by current terminology: the terms
mother cell, daughter cell, generation, cohort (a group of individuals of nearly equal age) etc. are frequently used in cell biology.
In this terminology, cell division means death of the dividing (mother)
cell and simultaneous birth of two daughters.

In the process of cell division called mitosis, all the genetic material of the mother is transmitted to each of the daughters. (Only
the germ cells in sexual reproduction are produced by another type
of division, where the genetic material is halved). However, the iden-

tity of genetic information does not exclude diversity of the cyto-
plasm, and the progeny of a single cell may exhibit a great variety
of functional types. In fact, a single cell, the fertilized egg, is
the origin of all the different cell types which constitute the adult
organism. Embryonic development is an extremely well-organized process
of proliferation, differentiation, and migration of cells. Differentiation means a gradual change of morphology and cell metabolism from
generation to generation. The endpoint of each differentiation pathway
is a mature cell that has a definite task in a complex system of division of labor. These end cells or functional cells have lost the
proliferative capacity. They are sterile.

A tissue may grow as a result of an increase in the size of the cells
or in the amount of intercellular substance. However, these processes
are of secondary importance in comparison with growth caused by an
increase of cell number, i.e. cell proliferation. The tissues of the
adult have ceased to grow, because there is no more proliferation (as
in the nervous system) or because there is an equilibrium of cell proliferation and cell loss. This occurs in the renewal tissues, which
contain a subpopulation of stem cells, i.e. undifferentiated cells
with nearly unlimited capacity of proliferation. In equilibrium, one
half of the cells born by the proliferating stem cells become again
stem cells and one half are committed to differentiation. The latter
have to migrate and pass through several maturation stages until they
reach the functional stage, and after a certain time in the functional
stage they die (Fig.1). A fraction of the stem cells are in a resting
state, like a reserve that can be activated when abnormal cell loss
has disturbed equilibrium.

This will be illustrated by an example. The blood cells (erythrocytes,
leukocytes, thrombocytes), which are completely different with respect
to morphology and function, are differentiated end cells originating

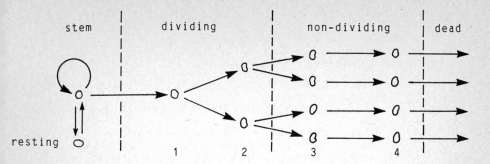

Fig.1: A tree diagram of a cell system with 4 maturation stages. The proliferative capacity is lost at the 3rd stage. The last stage is the functional stage.

from a single pool of pluripotent stem cells in the red bone marrow. The transit time through the maturation stages of erythro-, leuko-, and thrombocytes differs considerably between the 3 cell types, the same as the life time of the functional cells. Therefore the loss of stem cells or cells of early maturation stages (e.g. as a side effect of cytostatic treatment) becomes apparent at different times in the count of the respective end cell types. The delay is 3-7 days for leukocytes, 10-14 days for thrombocytes and 6-8 weeks for erythrocytes. A feedback regulation mechanism restores the normal state (see Sec.7 of Chap.III). Mathematical models of this mechanism have been studied by Wichmann (1984).

The concept of cell population, which is crucial in this monograph, is a mixture of the statistical and the biological concepts of population or species. A statistical population may be defined by any property that a member of the population should possess. The population of erythrocytes of a vertebrate is well defined in a statistical sense, because it is a set of cells with common morphological and functional properties; but it lacks the essential property of a species to support itself by proliferation. On the other hand, the concept of species as applied to sexually reproducing animals and plants cannot be applied to cells. We define a cell population to be a population of cells in the statistical sense, which is capable of supporting itself by proliferation. Examples of cell populations are:

1) the liver cells, 2) the erythrocytes together with their stem cells and all intermediate maturation stages, 3) a clone of immunocompetent T-cells according to the clonal selection theory of Burnet (Burnet, 1976), 4) a tumor.

Cell population kinetics (briefly: cell kinetics) is the investigation of the structure, the proliferative activity and the growth of cell populations. For example, a cell kinetic study of the cell system represented in Fig.1 should determine the transit time of cells through the different stages. In the absence of growth and of any perturbation (e.g. by irradiation or chemotherapy), the transit time is related to the input per time unit and the number n_c of cells according to the formula

$$n_c = \text{input} \cdot \text{transit time} \qquad (1.1)$$

The input to each stage is equal to or twice the input of the foregoing stage, depending on whether or not division takes place. Suppose, for example, that the stem cells in Fig.1 produce a net number of 10^6 cells/day, and let the transit time through stage i be t_i days (i=1,2,3,4), then the numbers of cells at the 4 maturation stages are $n_1=t_1 10^6$, $n_2=2t_2 10^6$, $n_3=4t_3 10^6$, $n_4=4t_4 10^6$. The simplicity of these formulae is due to the fact that the cell population is in a steady state. When the population is growing, more complicated formulae must be used.

It is supposed that a normal proliferating cell of an adult organism is sensitive to a certain biochemical signal controlling its proliferation. The chalone theory postulates that the proliferative activity of stem cells is inhibited by a specific protein (the chalone) produced by the end cells descending from them (see Houck, 1976). The more end cells there are, the more chalone is produced; hence there is a negative feedback, which prevents excessive growth.

The sensitivity to growth controlling signals must depend on the genome of each cell. When as many cell divisions occur as in the bone marrow or in the intestinal epithelium, there is a real risk that a cell will lose the gene of proliferation control by mutation. All descendants of that cell will have the same genetic defect, and an ever growing population of poorly differentiated cells, a tumor, will arise unless the immune surveillance of the body eliminates the degenerated cells from the beginning. Another theory suggests that the origin of cancer, especially of leukemias, is a failure of differentiation, and it proposes the induction of differentiation as a new way of therapy (Sachs 1986).

2. The cell cycle

The cell cycle is the process between two subsequent cell divisions.
A great deal of our knowledge about the cell cycle has been reported
in an article by Baserga (1981). The most important facts are summa-
rized in a survey article by Bertuzzi et al. (1981): "The cell cycle
is an ordered sequence of biochemical events leading up to cell division (mitosis). The essential aspect of this process is that each
daughter cell must have the same quantity of DNA of the mother; so
the mother's DNA has to be replicated before division. The cycle can
be divided into four phases, called G_1, S, G_2 and M. In G_1 (the gap
period), RNA and proteins are synthesized in preparation for the DNA
replication that takes place in S (the synthetic period); then the
cell progresses through G_2, which is a second gap period, and finally
enters mitosis (M). Each daughter cell can again traverse the cycle,
or can shift to a quiescent state during which cells do not divide for
long periods. It is still a subject of debate whether these quiescent
cells have entered a qualitatively different phase, called G_0, or a
prolonged G_1. Quiescent cells, however, retain for a long time the
ability to recycle under proper conditions or stimuli." The cycle
events and the possible states of noncycling cells are represented
in Fig.2.

During mitosis the chromosomes become visible and produce characteristic "mitotic figures". Four stages of mitosis can be distinguished
optically: prophase, metaphase, anaphase, telophase. But mitosis is
the unique phase of the cycle with characteristic visible features.
Therefore the distinction between S-phase and the "gap" phases was
not possible before the early 50's, when H^3-Thymidine became available for experiments. Thymidine is a specific precursor of DNA, such

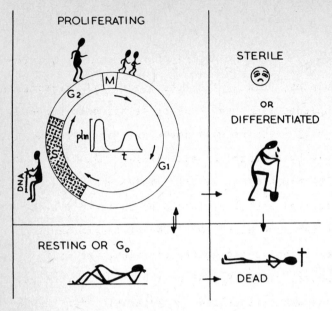

Fig.2.: A cartoon
representation of
the cell cycle and
of state transitions.
During S-phase the
cell is knitting
the double helix
of DNA. (From Dene-
kamp, Cell Kinetics
and Cancer Therapy,
1982. Courtesy of
Charles C. Thomas,
Publisher, Spring-
field, Illinois).

that only cells synthesizing DNA become labelled with H^3 (tritium)
when a cell population is exposed to H^3-Thymidine. Labelled cells are
recognized with the autoradiographic method (see Chap.II), but weakly
labelled cells may fail to be detected, due to background noise. Therefore, Shackney (1973) argued that labelling experiments cannot prove
that DNA-synthesis is totally absent during the gap phases. Nicolini
(1975) answered him with a comprehensive apologia of the theory of
discrete phases.

A part of Chap.II will be devoted to the determination of the length
of phases. Mitosis has a duration of about 1 h, S-phase may vary between 8 and 20 h depending on cell type, G_2 is always short (less than
4 h); but G_1 may exceed 40 h. The terms phase length, phase duration,
and transit time (through phase φ) are synonymous.

The duration of the cell cycle is called the cycle time or generation
time. Often it is assumed that the cycle time has a unique value T_c
for all cells of a cell population. But there may be a broad range

of cycle times in the population, and several types of distribution have been proposed to describe the distribution of cycle times. It is difficult to decide which of these gives the best fit to all the known data.

Cell age is defined in the same way as the age of an organism: the time since birth. But the time since birth is not always an exact indicator of position in the cell cycle, because the duration of phases may vary. Therefore the concept of maturity or functional age is also used (Rubinow, 1968). This concept is related to the maturation process that is going on during the cell cycle. Two cells that are leaving the S-phase simultaneously are of equal functional age, although they may have been born at different times. When ambiguity is possible, the time since birth will be called chronological age. A cell population is called synchronized if all its members are of nearly equal functional age. Synchronized cells in vitro can be obtained by several techniques (Grdina et al., 1984, Nias and Fox, 1971), and are used in many cell kinetic experiments.

3. The simple model of tumor growth

Let us look again at Fig.1 and try to describe the picture in purely kinetic terms. If we forget for a moment the resting cells, then there are $n_0 + n_1$ cells (stem + stage 1) that produce 2 dividing cells at each division, and n_2 dividing cells that produce only non-dividing cells. We define the division factor α as the average number of dividing cells rising from one cell division. In the present case we have

$$\alpha = \frac{2n_0 + 2n_1 + 0 \cdot n_2}{n_0 + n_1 + n_2} .$$

If the cycle time of all proliferating cells is equal and if cell production and cell loss are in equilibrium, then according to eq.(1.1) $n_0 = 2n_1 = n_2$ and hence $\alpha = 1$.

The simple model of tumor growth will be obtained from the model of Fig.1, if the purely kinetic facts are isolated and if α is allowed to take any value between 1 and 2. There are now 3 types of cells, which we call P-cells (proliferating), G_0-cells (resting) and Q-cells (sterile). G_0-cells are not sterile and can re-enter the cell cycle. The term stem cell no longer is used, since we do not consider differentiation. We assume that cell division is random and that a P-cell divides with probability $\delta \Delta t$ in a small time interval Δt. It then can be shown that the fraction of P-cells that have not divided in the interval $[t, t+t_1]$ is $e^{-\delta t_1}$. This means that some P-cells cannot be distinguished from resting cells during a finite time of observation. Therefore, if resting cells are considered as proliferating cells with a prolonged cycle time, it is sufficient to consider only P-cells (including G_0-cells) and Q-cells (Fig.3).

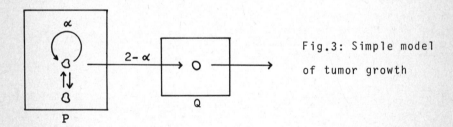

Fig.3: Simple model of tumor growth

The following terminology will be used:

$P(t)$	number of P-cells at time t	
$Q(t)$	number of Q-cells at time t	
α	division factor (average number of P-cells born per cell division)	
δ	rate of cell division (as defined previously)	
λ	rate of loss of Q-cells	

We will always assume α, δ and λ to be constant and $1 \le \alpha \le 2$.

With $N(t) = P(t) + Q(t)$, the total number of cells, the "proliferative fraction" $PF(t)$ is defined by

$$PF(t) = \frac{P(t)}{N(t)}$$

The term "growth fraction" also is used, but can be misleading in suggesting P is growing and Q not.

It now is possible to derive a pair of differential equations to describe the growth of P and Q. During a short time, from t to $t+\Delta t$, there are $\delta \Delta t\, P(t)$ cell divisions, and $\lambda \Delta t\, Q(t)$ cells are lost. α P-cells and $(2-\alpha)$ Q-cells are born, and 1 P-cell vanishes, per division. This leads to the equations

$$P(t+\Delta t) - P(t) = (\alpha-1)\,\delta\, P(t)\, \Delta t$$
$$Q(t+\Delta t) - Q(t) = (2-\alpha)\,\delta\, P(t)\, \Delta t - \lambda\, Q(t)\, \Delta t$$

If we write

$$\sigma = (\alpha-1)\delta \qquad\qquad \tau = (2-\alpha)\delta \qquad\qquad (3.1)$$

and let $\Delta t \to 0$, we get the differential equations

$$\frac{dP}{dt} = \sigma P \qquad\qquad (3.2a)$$

$$\frac{dQ}{dt} = \tau P - \lambda Q \qquad\qquad (3.2b)$$

The system (2a/b) is linear, and its solution is obtained easily. But primary interest is in the behavior of PF, and one can derive directly from the definition of PF and from (2a/b) that

$$\frac{d}{dt}\left(\frac{1}{PF}\right) = \tau - (\lambda+\sigma)\left(\frac{1}{PF} - 1\right)$$

Therefore, from any initial value,

$$\frac{1}{PF} = \frac{1}{PF_\infty} + \left(\frac{1}{PF(0)} - \frac{1}{PF_\infty}\right) e^{-(\lambda+\sigma)t} \qquad\qquad (3.3)$$

in which

$$PF_\infty = (\lambda+\sigma)/(\lambda+\sigma+\tau) \qquad\qquad (3.4)$$

The special case $\lambda=0$ and $\sigma=0$ (i.e., $\alpha=1$) represents a cell population with constant P, linearly increasing Q, and PF decreasing asymptotically to zero; it will not be treated henceforth.

If $PF(0) = PF_\infty$, PF will not change, although P and Q will both be increasing at the common rate σ; if $PF(0) \neq PF_\infty$, this pattern of growth still represents the asymptotic behavior of the population.

From arbitrary starting conditions $P(0) = P_0$, $Q(0) = Q_0$, one can derive the value for the total population size at time t by using the formulae $P(t) = P_0 e^{\sigma t}$ and (3.3), since

$$N(t) = P(t)/PF(t).$$

In particular, this leads to

$$N(t) = P_0\{\frac{1}{PF_\infty} e^{\sigma t} + (\frac{1}{PF(0)} - \frac{1}{PF_\infty}) e^{-\lambda t}\} \qquad (3.5)$$

Thus, for $\lambda > 0$ and t large, the total number of cells does not depend on the number of Q-cells at t=0. This fact may be written more precisely in the following way:

$$\lim_{t \to \infty} N(t)e^{-\sigma t} = P_0/PF_\infty. \qquad (3.6)$$

So far we have assumed that only Q-cells are subject to loss. Now suppose that P-cells are lost at a rate λ_P and denote the loss rate of Q-cells with λ_Q. Then the equations (2a/b) become

$$\frac{dP}{dt} = (\sigma - \lambda_P)P \qquad (3.7a)$$

$$\frac{dQ}{dt} = \tau P - \lambda_Q Q \qquad (3.7b)$$

and hence, in eq. (3), (4), (5) and (6) σ is to be replaced by $\sigma-\lambda_P$ and λ by λ_Q, in particular we have now

$PF_\infty = (\lambda_Q - \lambda_P + \sigma)/(\lambda_Q - \lambda_P + \sigma + \tau)$. In the special case $\lambda_P = \lambda_Q$ we obtain using eq. (1) and deleting the subscript ∞,

$$PF = \alpha - 1 \qquad\qquad (3.8)$$

This equation is used very frequently in cell kinetic calculations.

In this and all the following cell kinetic models, the rate of exponential growth shall be denoted with ρ. In order to calculate ρ we sum eq. (7a) and (7b) and divide through $N = P + Q$, which gives

$$(dN/dt)/N = (\sigma + \tau - \lambda_P)PF - \lambda_Q(1 - PF)$$

In the state of exponential growth we have $dN/dt = \rho N$ and $PF = PF_\infty$. Therefore, according to eq. (1) we obtain

$$\rho = \delta\,PF_\infty - \{\lambda_P\,PF_\infty + \lambda_Q(1 - PF_\infty)\} \qquad\qquad (3.9)$$

This equation shows how the rate of exponential growth depends on the rate of cell division, on the proliferative fraction and on the cell loss rates.

For the special case $\lambda_P = 0$, Steel (1968) has defined the cell loss factor Φ as the ratio of cell loss to net production of cells: $\Phi = (\lambda_Q Q)/(\delta P)$. It must be emphasized that Φ is constant, if and only if PF is constant. This will be supposed in the sequel, and the subscript ∞ will be omitted. Now, $\lambda_P = 0$ and $dP/dt = \rho P$ imply $\rho = \sigma = (\alpha-1)\delta$, and from eq. (9) we deduce $\rho = \delta\,PF - \lambda_Q(1 - PF)$. Therefore, since $1 - PF = Q/(P + Q)$, we obtain

$$\alpha - 1 = PF\left(1 - \frac{\lambda_Q}{\delta}\,\frac{Q}{P}\right) = PF(1 - \Phi)$$

and hence

$$PF = \frac{\alpha - 1}{1 - \Phi} \qquad\qquad (3.10)$$

This equation has been proved for a different pattern of cell loss by Steel (1977). A similar formula, which includes loss of P-cells, can be derived assuming an arbitrary distribution of cycle times (Knolle 1983b).

In the previous model we have assumed that the parameters σ, τ and λ are constant. A two-compartment model, in which σ depends on P, has been studied by Eisen (1977) with a view to modelling the breakdown of normal growth control and subsequent unlimited growth.

4. The extended model of tumor growth

In the preceding section we have assumed that resting cells (G_0-cells) can be considered as P-cells with a cycle time much longer than the interval of observation. This would imply that the proportion of resting cells depends on the distribution of cycle times and on the experimental design. This problem can be overcome by defining the compartment of Q-cells in such a way that it includes resting and sterile cells and that Q-cells can return to the compartment of P-cells. The transition of cells from the resting state to the proliferative state is very important in radio- and chemotherapy of cancer where it is called "recruitment of resting cells into the cell cycle". In cancer therapy, recruitment is induced artificially and the flow of recruited cells may change abruptly with time. This will be discussed in Chapter III. For the moment we will consider only the constant flow of resting cells into the pool of proliferating cells, which has been observed in some normal cell populations (Korr et al. 1983).

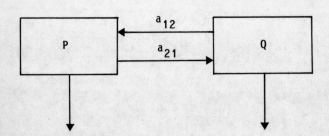

Fig.4: Extended model of tumor growth

Starting from equations (3.7a/b), we could write

$$\frac{dP}{dt} = (\sigma - \lambda_P)P + \gamma Q$$

$$\frac{dQ}{dt} = \tau P - (\lambda_Q + \gamma)Q$$

where γQ is the number of cells which pass from Q to P in the time unit. But we prefer to change the whole terminology and write

$$\frac{dP}{dt} = a_{11}P + a_{12}Q \qquad (4.1a)$$

$$\frac{dQ}{dt} = a_{21}P + a_{22}Q \qquad (4.1b)$$

where $a_{12}, a_{21} > 0$, $a_{22} < 0$. a_{11} is a lumped parameter resulting from proliferation minus cell loss and transition. a_{12} and a_{21} are the rates of transition from Q to P and from P to Q. Again we define a "proliferative fraction" by $PF(t) = P(t)\{P(t) + Q(t)\}^{-1}$; but the following calculations will be in terms of $R(t) = Q(t)/P(t)$. From eq. (1a/b) we derive

$$\frac{dR}{dt} = a_{21} + (a_{22} - a_{11})R - a_{12}R^2. \qquad (4.2)$$

Let $r > 0$ and $s < 0$ be the solutions of the equation

$$a_{21} + (a_{22} - a_{11})x - a_{12}x^2 = 0 . \qquad (4.3)$$

Then

$$\frac{dR}{dt} = -a_{12}(R-r)(R-s)$$

$$-a_{12}(r-s)t = \int \left(\frac{1}{R-r} - \frac{1}{R-s}\right) dR$$

$$\frac{R(t)-r}{R(t)-s} = c \, \exp\{-a_{12}(r-s)t\}$$

where $c = (R_0-r)/(R_0-s)$ and $R_0 = R(0)$. Therefore we obtain

$$R(t) = \frac{r(R_0-s) - s(R_0-r) \exp(-a_{12}(r-s)t)}{(R_0-s) - (R_0-r) \exp(-a_{12}(r-s)t)} \qquad (4.4)$$

which replaces eq. (3.4). Note that $R(t) \rightarrow r$ as $t \rightarrow \infty$ and that

$$a_{12}(r-s) = \sqrt{(a_{11}-a_{22})^2 + 4a_{12}a_{21}} \qquad (4.5)$$

Thus the rate of convergence is an increasing function of the rates of flow between the compartments, and it reduces to $a_{11}-a_{22}$ or $\sigma+\lambda$ in the case $a_{12}=0$ (simple model of tumor growth). Now, if $R_0 = r$ then $R(t) = r$ for all t, and $P' = (a_{11}+a_{12}r)P$, $Q' = (a_{21}r^{-1}+a_{22})Q$. Since r satisfies eq. (3), which may be written $a_{21}r^{-1}+a_{22} = a_{11}+a_{12}r$, both P and Q are growing exponentially with rate ρ, where

$$\rho = a_{11} + a_{12}r \qquad \text{or} \qquad \rho = a_{21}r^{-1} + a_{22} \qquad (4.6)$$

So far, the situation is rather similar to that of the preceding section: PF(t) approaches a unique equilibrium value $PF_\infty = 1/(1+r)$, which entails exponential growth of both compartments. But there is an important difference if we ask for the total number of cells. In fact, eq. (3.5a) has to be replaced by

$$\lim_{t \rightarrow \infty} N(t)e^{-\rho t} = c(P_0,Q_0)/PF_\infty \qquad (4.7)$$

where

$$c(P_0,Q_0) = \frac{a_{21}P_0 + a_{12}rQ_0}{a_{21} + a_{12}r^2} \qquad (4.8)$$

This follows from eq. (1.4), Theorem 2, and eq. (1.9) of the Appendix. Therefore, the ultimate number of cells depends on both P_0 and Q_0 when $a_{12} > 0$.

3. Cell age distributions and phase indices

The preceding analysis did not consider the age and the phases of the cell cycle of proliferating cells. This gap will be filled in the present and the following sections.

The S-phase index I_S is the fraction of cells in S with respect to all cells; indices of G_1, G_2, and M are defined analogously. We shall derive expressions for the phase indices in terms of the phase durations and other kinetic parameters.

Let us introduce a function $u(a,t)$ of the two variables a (age) and t (time) with the following property:

For any pair of numbers a_1, a_2 $(0 \leq a_1 < a_2)$, the integral

$$\int_{a_1}^{a_2} u(a,t) \, da$$

is the number of cells with age between a_1 and a_2 at time t.

If $a_2 - a_1$ is very small, then we may approximate the integral by $(a_2 - a_1)u(a_1,t)$.

On the other hand, if we extend the interval of integration from 0 to ∞ (avoiding the problem of guessing an upper limit of cell age), then we obtain the total number of cells at time t:

$$N(t) = \int_{0}^{\infty} u(a,t) \, da$$

The function u(a,t) is called the cell age <u>density</u> at time t. The cell age <u>distribution</u> η(a,t) is now defined by

$$\eta(a,t) = \frac{u(a,t)}{N(t)}$$

According to this definition $\int_{a_1}^{a_2} \eta(a,t)\, da$ is the fraction of cells with age between a_1 and a_2 at time t.

Now we apply these concepts to the simple model of tumor growth as outlined in Section 3. Since a cell synthesising DNA is surely a P-cell, the decision whether a cell will continue the cycle or drop to the resting state must be made before the beginning of S-phase. In the evaluation of the experiments to be discussed later (e.g. labelling of cells in S-phase) it makes no difference, whether this decision is assumed in late or in early G_1-phase or immediately after mitosis. The last assumption facilitates the mathematical treatment and will be adopted here.

In this section we suppose that all P-cells complete the cycle with uniform cycle time T_C and phase durations T_{G_1}, T_S, T_{G_2}, T_M. Remember that in the simple model of tumor growth no Q-cells re-enter the cycle. Now let u(a,t) be the age density and η(a,t) the age distribution of P-cells. Since a cell that has age a at time t has been born at time t-a, we have

$$u(a,t) = u(0,t-a) \qquad (0 \le a \le T_C) \qquad (5.1)$$

Every P-cell that has reached the age T_C divides and produces 2 daughter cells of age 0, namely α P-cells and (2-α) Q-cells in the mean. Hence

$$u(0,t) = \alpha u(T_C,t) \qquad (5.2)$$

and after division through $P(t) = \int_0^\infty u(a,t)da$

$$n(0,t) = \alpha n(T_C,t) \qquad (5.2a)$$

The equations (1), (2) and (2a) are satisfied by any age density (distribution) under the conditions assumed. Now we look for the special age distributions which are constant in time, i.e. we suppose that $n(a,t)$ is a function of a alone, $n(a,t) = A(a)$ or

$$u(a,t) = A(a)P(t) \qquad (5.3)$$

At first we insert eq.(3) into eq.(1) and get

$$A(a)P(t) = A(0)P(t-a) \qquad (5.4)$$

with the special case

$$A(a)P(0) = A(0)P(-a) \qquad (5.4a)$$

From eq.(4) and eq.(4a) we get easily

$$P(t-a) = P(t)A(a)A(0)^{-1} = P(t)P(-a)P(0)^{-1}$$

This equation must hold for any t and for $0 \leq a \leq T_C$. The only mathematical function with this property is the exponential; hence $P(t) = P(0)e^{\rho t}$, where the constant ρ is still unknown. Inserting this function into eq.(4) we get

$$A(a)e^{\rho t} = A(0)e^{\rho(t-a)}$$

$$A(a) = A(0)e^{-\rho a} \qquad (0 \leq a \leq T_C) \qquad (5.5)$$

During one cycle time T_C, the number of P-cells increases by the factor α, hence $\exp(\rho T_C) = \alpha$ or

$$\rho = \frac{\log \alpha}{T_C} \qquad (5.6)$$

The function A(a) is called the age distribution and ρ the rate of exponential ("log phase") growth. The age density of exponential growth can be written in the form

$$u(a,t) = c\, e^{\rho(t-a)} \qquad (5.7)$$

where $c = A(0)P(0)$.

Equation (6) is sometimes written in the equivalent form

$$\alpha e^{-\rho T_C} = 1 \qquad (5.6a)$$

and can be derived from eq.(2a), too.

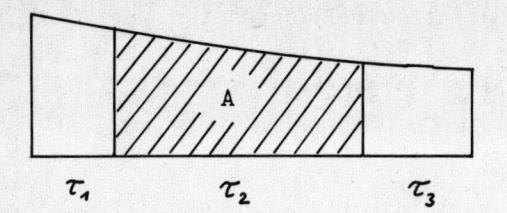

Fig.5: Fraction of cells with age between τ_1 and $\tau_1+\tau_2$

Let τ_1, τ_2, τ_3 be nonnegative numbers with sum T_C. The fraction of P-cells with age between τ_1 and $\tau_1+\tau_2$ is the ratio of the shaded area A to the whole area B under the exponential curve in fig.5. Now we have

$$A = \int_{\tau_1}^{\tau_1+\tau_2} e^{-\rho a}\, da = \frac{1}{\rho} e^{-\rho\tau_1}(1-e^{-\rho\tau_2})$$

$$B = \int_{0}^{\tau_1+\tau_2+\tau_3} e^{-\rho a}\, da = \frac{1}{\rho}(1-e^{-\rho(\tau_1+\tau_2+\tau_3)})$$

Multiplying each member of the ratio A/B with $e^{\rho(\tau_1+\tau_3)}e^{\rho\tau_2}$ we get

$$\frac{A}{B} = \frac{e^{\rho\tau_3}(e^{\rho\tau_2}-1)}{e^{\rho(\tau_1+\tau_2+\tau_3)}-1} \qquad (5.8)$$

This expression will be reduced to a surprisingly simple form, using he approximation

$$e^x - 1 \approx x \, e^{\frac{1}{2}x} \tag{5.9}$$

hich is suggested by the expansion

$$e^x - 1 = e^{\frac{1}{2}x}(e^{\frac{1}{2}x} - e^{-\frac{1}{2}x})$$

$$= e^{\frac{1}{2}x}(x + \frac{1}{24}x^3 + \dots)$$

It can be shown that the relative error of this approximation is less than 0.02, if x is between 0 and log 2. This condition is satisfied if we take $x = \rho\tau_2$ or $x = \rho(\tau_1 + \tau_2 + \tau_3) = \rho T_C$, since $\rho \leq \log 2/T_C$. Applying eq.(9) to both members of the ratio in eq.(8) we get

$$\frac{A}{B} \approx \frac{\tau_2}{\tau_1 + \tau_2 + \tau_3} \, e^{\frac{1}{2}\rho(\tau_3 - \tau_1)} \tag{5.8a}$$

with an error less than 0.02. This equation which applies also when the sum of τ_1, τ_2 and τ_3 is less than T_C, is very suggestive because of its symmetry. Now we deduce an equivalent formula, using $\tau_1 + \tau_2 + \tau_3 = T_C$ and $\exp(\rho T_C) = \alpha$. From (8) and (9) we get

$$\frac{A}{B} = \frac{1}{\alpha - 1} \, e^{\rho\tau_3}(e^{\rho\tau_2} - 1)$$

$$\frac{A}{B} \approx \frac{1}{\alpha - 1} \, \rho\tau_2 \, e^{\rho(\frac{1}{2}\tau_2 + \tau_3)} \tag{5.8b}$$

Inserting $\rho = \log \alpha/T_C$, this can be written

$$\frac{A}{B} \approx \frac{\log \alpha}{\alpha - 1} \, \frac{\tau_2}{T_C} \, \alpha^{(\frac{1}{2}\tau_2 + \tau_3)/T_C} \tag{5.8c}$$

Of course, these expressions have to be multiplied by PF, if the fraction with respect to the whole population is considered. In particular, for the S-phase index I_S we have

$$I_S = \frac{PF}{\alpha - 1} e^{\rho T_3} (e^{\rho T_S} - 1) \qquad (5.10)$$

$$I_S \approx PF \frac{T_S}{T_C} e^{\frac{1}{2}\rho(T_3 - T_1)} \qquad (5.10a)$$

$$I_S \approx PF \frac{T_S}{T_C} \frac{\log \alpha}{\alpha - 1} \alpha^r \qquad (5.10c)$$

where $T_1 = T_{G_1}$, $T_3 = T_{G_2} + T_M$ and $r = (\frac{1}{2}T_S + T_3)/T_C$. Hence, the approximation $I_S \approx PF(T_S/T_C)$ used in most cell kinetic studies is quite good, if T_3 is near T_1. The correction factor appearing in eq. (10c) is plotted in Fig.6 as a function of α for various values of r. It is close to 1 for all values of α, if r = 1/2, i.e. if the middle of the S-phase coincides with the middle of the cycle or if $T_1 = T_3$.

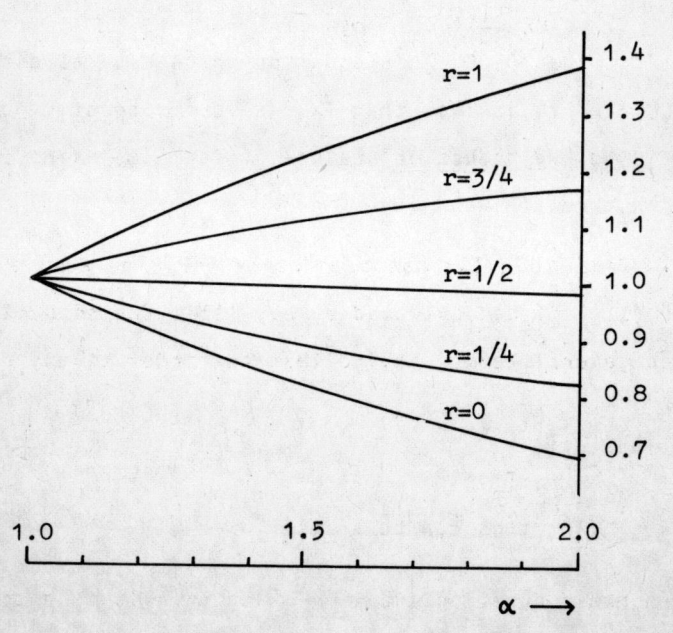

Fig.6: Correction factor $\alpha^r \log \alpha/(\alpha-1)$ for various values of r and $1 \leq \alpha \leq 2$. The case r=1/2 leads to the approximation (5.11).

ncidentally we get from Fig.6 the useful formula

$$\frac{\log x}{x-1} \approx x^{-\frac{1}{2}} \qquad (1 \leq x \leq 2) \qquad (5.11)$$

n order to calculate the mitotic index I_M we take $\tau_3=0$, $\tau_2=T_M$, $\tau_1=T_C-T_M$ in eq.(8a) and get

$$I_M \approx PF \frac{T_M}{T_C} e^{-\frac{1}{2}\rho(T_C-T_M)}$$

Since ρT_M is small and $e^{\rho T_C} = \alpha$, we obtain

$$I_M \approx PF \frac{T_M}{T_C} \alpha^{-\frac{1}{2}} \qquad (5.12a)$$

From eq.(8b) we get in the same way

$$I_M \approx PF \frac{1}{\alpha-1} \rho T_M \exp(\tfrac{1}{2} \rho T_M) \qquad (5.12b)$$

and from eq.(8c)

$$I_M \approx PF \frac{\log \alpha}{\alpha-1} \frac{T_M}{T_C} \qquad (5.12c)$$

where the factor $\exp(\tfrac{1}{2}\rho T_M/T_C)$ has been neglected. The equivalence of eqs. (12a) and (12c) is demonstrated by eq. (11). The situation may be described in general terms, saying that the index of any phase φ is given by

$$I_\varphi = PF \frac{T_\varphi}{T_C} k_\varphi \qquad (5.13)$$

where T_φ is the phase duration and $k_\varphi = \alpha^r \log \alpha/(\alpha-1)$ is a correction factor. For any phase and any value of α k_φ can be read from Fig.6, if r is given the appropriate value, namely:

$$r = (\tfrac{1}{2}T_1 + T_S + T_3)/T_C \qquad \text{for phase } G_1$$

$$r = (\tfrac{1}{2}T_S + T_3)/T_C \qquad \text{for phase } S$$

$$r = (\tfrac{1}{2}T_{G_2} + T_M)/T_C \qquad \text{for phase } G_2$$

$$r = 0 \qquad \text{for phase } M$$

All equations of this section have been derived under the assumption of uniform cycle time and phase durations. It will be shown later (Sec.7) that this assumption is not necessary.

6. The general model with distributed cycle time

If all present and future cells of a population had the same cycle time, then the age distribution of exponential growth would be an exceptional case. A clone, i.e. a population of descendants of a single cell, would never reach this age distribution and would have a mitotic index oscillating between 0 and 1. Such a state of synchrony with respect to the cell cycle is sometimes observed in a disturbed cell population, but after a due time of recovery the population attains a state of asynchronous proliferation in which the mitotic index is constant. Therefore, it is necessary to introduce a more realistic model of cell populations with a distribution of cycle times. In Sec.3 we already admitted a range of cycle times from 0 to ∞, but the distribution was very special. In the present section the general framework of the simple model with the distinction of P- and Q-cells is retained, but the cycle time is thought to be a random variable with an arbitrary probability distribution.

Since this section is rather long and charged with mathematics, a brief summary is given now. It is shown that an initially synchronous population approaches ultimately a stable age distribution, which admits exponential growth. This process of decay of synchrony exhibits damped oscillations of the phase indices with a period near the mean cycle time $\overline{T}$ and a damping factor that depends on the variance of the cycle time. The rate of exponential growth ρ is the unique real solution of the "characteristic equation" (6.8), which generalizes eq. (5.6).

In Sec.3 we assumed that a cell divided with probability $\delta\Delta t$ in a small time interval of length Δt and that δ was constant. Now we start with the same assumption, but let δ depend on age. Furthermore, we allow that P-cells are lost at a constant rate without division. A P-cell is said to survive if neither loss nor division has occurred.

The following denotations will be used:

u(a,t)   age density of P-cells

v(a,t)   age density of Q-cells

φ(a)   probability for P-cells to survive up to age a

ψ(a)   probability for Q-cells to survive up to age a

δ(a)   probability density for P-cells of age a to divide

α division factor for P-cells

λ_P, λ_Q rates of random loss of P-cells and Q-cells

Since it is assumed that no Q-cells reenter the cell cycle, the growth of the whole population depends exclusively on the kinetics of P-cells, i.e. on φ(a), δ(a), λ_P and α. Therefore, we will first study the relations between these parameters or functions and the age density of P-cells. The prefix "P" is omitted henceforth.

The age density at age 0, u(0,t), is called the birth density. u(a,t) can be calculated from birth density and survival probability through the equation

$$u(a,t) = u(0,t-a) \; \varphi(a) \qquad (a \geq 0) \qquad \qquad (6.1)$$

According to the definition of δ(a) and α we have

$$u(0,t) = \alpha \int_0^\infty u(a,t) \; \delta(a) \; da \qquad \qquad (6.2)$$

Obviously, these equations generalize eq.(5.1) and eq.(5.2).

The survival probability and the probability density of division satisfy

$$\varphi(0) = 1 \qquad \lim_{a \to \infty} \varphi(a) = 0 \qquad \int_0^\infty \delta(a)\ da = 1 \qquad (6.3a)$$

Given a cell of age a and a short time interval of length h, there are three possibilities: division, loss, or survival up to age a+h. The probabilities of these mutually exclusive events are $\delta(a)h$, $\lambda_p h$ and $1-\delta(a)h-\lambda_p h$. Hence

$$\varphi(a+h) = (1-\delta(a)h-\lambda_p h)\varphi(a)$$

and as $h \to 0$,

$$\varphi'(a) = -\delta(a)\ \varphi(a)-\lambda_p\varphi(a) \qquad (6.3b)$$

These relations will be used later.

Now suppose that we know u(a,0), i.e. the age density at time t=0. How can we calculate u(a,t) for t > 0? We consider first the case $a \ge t$, i.e. those cells which were present at time t=0, their age at t=0 being $a-t \ge 0$. For any two positive numbers $a_1 < a_2$, the conditional probability that a cell which has survived up to age a_1 will survive up to age a_2 is $\varphi(a_2)/\varphi(a_1)$. Therefore the fraction of cells of age a-t that survive up to age a is $\varphi(a)/\varphi(a-t)$, and consequently

$$u(a,t) = \frac{\varphi(a)}{\varphi(a-t)}\ u(a-t,0) \qquad (a \ge t) \qquad (6.1a)$$

In order to obtain u(a,t) for a < t, i.e. the density of cells born after t=0, we have to calculate the birth density u(0,t) for t > 0. After that it is easy to calculate u(a,t) with the help of eq.(1).

For convenience we write $B(t) = u(0,t)$ and split $B(t)$ into the birth densities of overlapping generations.

We define:

> generation 0, consisting of all cells living at t=0;
> generation i, consisting of all daughters of cells of
> generation i-1 (i=1,2,...);
> $g_i(t)$, the birth density of generation i (i=1,2,...).

A cell of generation 1 born at time t has a mother of age $a \geq t$, hence

$$g_1(t) = \alpha \int_t^\infty u(a,t)\delta(a)da. \tag{6.4}$$

A cell of generation i > 1 born at time t has a mother of age $a \leq t$, which has been born at time t-a in generation i-1 and survived up to age a; hence

$$g_i(t) = \alpha \int_0^t g_{i-1}(t-a)\varphi(a)\delta(a)da \qquad (i=2,3,...)$$

Now we define $B_n(t) = \sum_{i=1}^n g_i(t)$ and have

$$B_n(t) = g_1(t) + \sum_{i=2}^n g_i(t)$$

$$= g_1(t) + \sum_{i=2}^n \alpha \int_0^t g_{i-1}(t-a)\varphi(a)\delta(a)da$$

$$= g_1(t) + \alpha \int_0^t \varphi(a)\delta(a) \sum_{i=1}^{n-1} g_i(t-a)da$$

$$= g_1(t) + \int_0^t \alpha \, \varphi(a)\delta(a)B_{n-1}(t-a)da$$

ntroducing the "net maternity function"

$$k(a) = \alpha\delta(a)\varphi(a), \tag{6.5}$$

e obtain the set of recursive equations

$$B_1(t) = g_1(t)$$

$$B_n(t) = g_1(t) + \int_0^t B_{n-1}(t-a)k(a)da$$

t is a reasonable assumption that there is a lower limit $\tau > 0$ for the ycle time. This implies that cells of generation n are not born before $= (n-1)\tau$, or that $g_n(t) = 0$ and $B_n(t) = B_{n-1}(t) = B(t)$ for $t < (n-1)\tau$. f eq.(1a) is inserted into eq.(4), this equation becomes

$$g_1(t) = \int_t^\infty \frac{u(a-t,0)}{\varphi(a-t)} k(a) \, da \tag{6.4a}$$

herefore, for any $t > 0$, the birth density can be calculated recursive-y, if $\varphi(a)$, $k(a)$ and $u(a,0)$ for $a \geq 0$ are known. Then the age density (a,t) is easily obtained using eq.(1). Saying it in equivalent terms, he development of the cell population can be prognosticated, if the ivision factor, the probabilities of survival and division, and the ge distribution at t=0 are known.

n some population models, the lower limit of the cycle time is zero, nd consequently, at any time $t > 0$ an infinite number of generations re coexisting.

Nevertheless, the relations $\lim\limits_{n \to \infty} \int B_n = \int \lim\limits_{n \to \infty} B_n$ and $\lim\limits_{n \to \infty} B_n = B$ hold under fairly general conditions, and passing to the limit in the recursive equation yields

$$B(t) = g_1(t) + \int_0^t B(t-a)k(a)da \qquad (6.6)$$

This linear integral equation, the renewal or Lotka equation, has been the subject of extensive studies in the past. As already mentioned, it can be solved by iteration. But for some purposes it is more convenient to apply the Laplace transformation. This way has been exposed e.g. by Hoppensteadt (1975) or Keyfitz (1977) and leads to the following statements.

The birth density is given by the series

$$B(t) = \sum_{i=0}^{\infty} c_i e^{\lambda_i t} \qquad (6.7)$$

where c_0 is a real and the other c_i are pairwise conjugate complex numbers, and the same holds for the λ_i. The c_i depend on $u(a,0)$, the age distribution at $t=0$, and the λ_i are the roots of the "characteristic equation"

$$\int_0^{\infty} e^{-\lambda a} k(a) da = 1 \qquad (6.8)$$

and hence are independent of $u(a,0)$. This equation has a unique real root λ_0, which is greater than $\text{Re}(\lambda_i)$, the real part of λ_i, for $i=1,2,\ldots$ Conditions for the existence of infinitely many roots of eq. (8) have been established by Hadwiger (1939). In spite of the presence of complex numbers in eq. (7), the sum is always real (due to conjugate pairs) and may be written alternatively with real numbers in the form

$$B(t) = c_0 e^{\rho t} + \sum_{i=1}^{\infty} e^{\mu_i t} (a_i \cos \nu_i t + b_i \sin \nu_i t) \qquad (6.7a)$$

where $\rho = \lambda_0$ and μ_i (ν_i) is the real (imaginary) part of the i-th pair of conjugate complex roots of eq. (8). Similar statements are valid in the case of uniform cycle time T_C and no cell loss. This is a limiting case, where $\delta(a)$ is a "distribution" (Dirac function) that satisfies $\delta(a) = 0$ for $a \neq T_C$ and $\int_0^{\infty} \delta(a) \, da = 1$. The characteristic equation is

$$\alpha e^{-\lambda T_C} = 1$$

and has the real root $\rho = \log \alpha / T_C$ already quoted in eq. (5.6), and the complex roots

$$\mu_n + \nu_n i = \rho \pm n \frac{2\pi i}{T_C} \qquad n = 1, 2, \ldots$$

Hence in this case all roots have equal real part ρ and the sum in eq. (7a) becomes a Fourier series (i.e. a periodic function with period T_C) multiplied by $e^{\rho t}$. This implies for example that the curve of fractions of labelled mitoses is periodic (see Sec.5, Chap.II).

Now suppose that $k(a) > 0$ at least in a small interval, and let $\lambda = \mu + \nu i$ be a complex root of eq. (8). Then there is at least a subinterval where $\cos \nu a < 1$ and hence

$$1 = \int_0^{\infty} e^{-\mu a} \cos \nu a \, k(a) \, da < \int_0^{\infty} e^{-\mu a} k(a) \, da$$

But the real root ρ makes the right side equal to 1, therefore $\rho > \mu$, and so we deduce from eq. (7a)

$$B(t) e^{-\rho t} = c_0 + \sum_{i=1}^{\infty} e^{(\mu_i - \rho)t} (\ldots)$$

$$\lim_{t \to \infty} B(t)\, e^{-\rho t} = c_0 \qquad\qquad (6.9)$$

This limit relation holds for an arbitrary distribution of cycle times. But the question, how the limit is approached, cannot be answered without reference to a particular distribution.

In demography the fitting of a distribution to empirical data on fertility of women is called a graduation. The normal and the gamma distribution have been chosen by Lotka respectively by Wicksell, and a new distribution has been introduced for this purpose by Hadwiger. The roots of the characteristic equation associated with these distributions have been investigated, and a survey is given in the book of Keyfitz (1977). The imaginary part of the pair with the greatest real part is approximately $2\pi/\overline{T}$ ($\overline{T}$ = mean cycle time) in all three graduations.

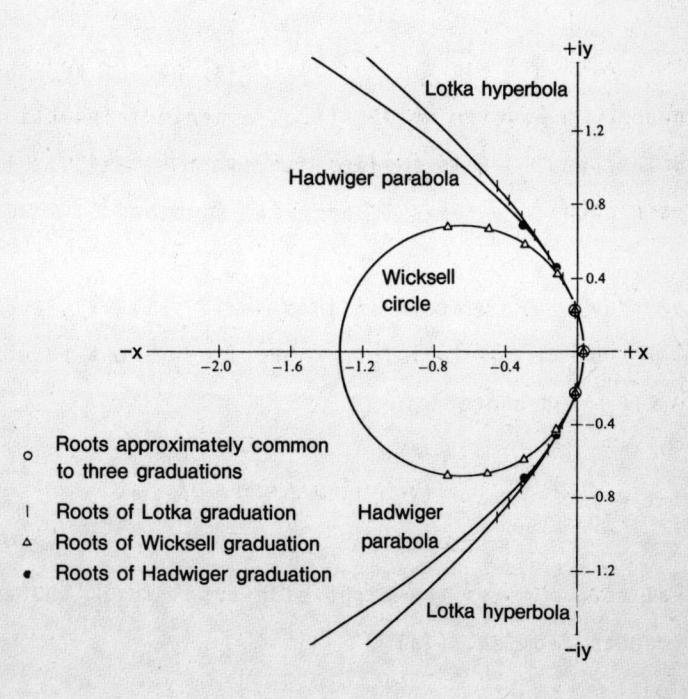

Fig.7: Roots of the characteristic equation in the complex plane
       (from Keyfitz, 1977)

The imaginary parts of the Hadwiger roots are close to multiples of $2\pi/\overline{T}$, while the real parts of the points on the Wicksell circle are rapidly decreasing (see Fig.7). Neither statement is true for the Lotka graduation. Thus, if we exclude the normal distribution from our consideration, the series in eq.(7a) contains only terms whose periodic factor oscillates with period $\overline{T}/n$ ($n=1,2,\ldots$) or whose exponential factor is neglegible compared with $e^{\rho t}$. It is well known that the superposition of oscillations of period $\overline{T}/n$ gives an oscillation of period $\overline{T}$. Therefore, the limit in eq.(9) is approached with damped oscillations of period $\overline{T}$.

Now we turn to the analogous statements for the age density and for the total number of P-cells. Using eq.(1), (7), and (9) we obtain

$$u(a,t) = \sum_{i=0}^{\infty} c_i e^{\lambda_i t} \varphi(a) e^{-\lambda_i a} \qquad (a < t) \qquad (6.10)$$

$$\lim_{t \to \infty} u(a,t) e^{-\rho t} = c_0 \, \varphi(a) e^{-\rho a} \qquad (6.11)$$

and, integrating over all ages,

$$\lim_{t \to \infty} P(t)e^{-\rho t} = c_0 \int_0^{\infty} \varphi(a) e^{-\rho a} \, da \qquad (6.12)$$

Applying partial integration, i.e.

$$\int_0^{\infty} \varphi'(a)e^{-\rho a} \, da = -1 + \rho \int_0^{\infty} \varphi(a)e^{-\rho a} \, da,$$

and then eq.(3b), (5), and (8), we obtain

$$\int_0^{\infty} \varphi(a)e^{-\rho a} \, da = \frac{\alpha-1}{\alpha(\rho+\lambda_p)} \qquad (6.13)$$

Since $\eta(a,t) = u(a,t)/P(t)$, we derive from eq.(11) and (12)

$$\lim_{t \to \infty} \eta(a,t) = A_o \varphi(a) e^{-\rho a} \qquad (A_o = \frac{\alpha(\rho + \lambda_p)}{\alpha - 1}) \qquad (6.14)$$

This result expresses the important stability property of the age distribution, and the function

$$A(a) = A_o \varphi(a) e^{-\rho a}$$

is therefore called the stable age distribution. It generalizes the age distribution of exponential growth considered in eq.(5.5). When the age distribution at $t = 0$ is stable, i.e. $u(a,0) = c_o \varphi(a) e^{-\rho a}$, then the coefficients c_i ($i=1,2,\ldots$) in eq.(10) are zero, and hence

$$u(a,t) = c_o e^{\rho t} \varphi(a) e^{-\rho a} \qquad (6.15)$$

in analogy to eq.(5.7). Therefore the stable age distribution entails exponential growth. When applied to an initially synchronous cell population, eq.(14) predicts the decay of synchrony, which is always observed in real cell populations.

Eq.(1) implies, that $u(a,t)$, $P(t)$ and $\eta(a,t)$ oscillate in the same way as the birth density. If this result is to be applied to observable quantities such as the labelling index, we are hampered by a little problem, which rises from the difference between chronological and functional age. This difference forbids it expressing a phase index by an integral of the form $\int_a^b \eta(x,t)\,dx$, where x is chronological age. But it is easy to get a correct expression in terms of the age distribution $\eta(x,t)$. Indeed, for each phase there is a function $F(a,b)$ of two variables, defined for $b \geq a \geq 0$, such that $F(a,b)\Delta a \Delta b$ is the fraction of cells that enter the phase with an age between a and $a + \Delta a$ and leave it between b and b+Δb. Then the phase index is given by

$$h(t) = \iint\limits_{a \leq b} \left(\int_a^b \eta(x,t)\, dx \right) F(a,b)\, da\, db$$

and this function exhibits a similar oscillation and limit behavior
as $\eta(x,t)$.

According to Bronk et al. (1968) the damping of oscillations obeys the
law

$$X_{max} - X_{avg} = Ae^{-\lambda t/\overline{T}} \tag{6.16}$$

where X_{avg} is the average and X_{max} is the peak of the quantity X (e.g.
the index of a phase) occurring at time t, and A and λ are constants.
For the gamma distribution they have derived $\lambda = 2\pi^2\sigma^2/\overline{T}^2$, where σ^2 is
the variance of the distribution.

To conclude this section, we treat the age density v(a,t) and the number Q(t) of Q-cells. Let $\psi(a)$ be the survival probability of Q-cells.
Then we have the analogue of eq.(1)

$$v(a,t) = v(0,t-a)\psi(a) \qquad (a \geq 0) \tag{6.17}$$

The birth densities of P- and Q-cells are related by the equation

$$u(0,t) = (\alpha/2)\{u(0,t) + v(0,t)\}$$

because $\alpha/2$ is the fraction of P-cells among the new-born cells. Hence
$v(0,t) = (2/\alpha-1)B(t)$, and therefore, using eq.(9) and (17), we obtain

$$\lim_{t \to \infty} v(a,t)e^{-\rho t} = c_0 \frac{2-\alpha}{\alpha} \psi(a)\, e^{-\rho a} \tag{6.18}$$

$$\lim_{t \to \infty} Q(t)e^{-\rho t} = c_0 \frac{2-\alpha}{\alpha} \int_0^\infty \psi(a) e^{-\rho a} da \qquad (6.19)$$

Now the limit of the proliferative fraction can be calculated, using eq.(12), (13), and (19). The result is (Knolle, 1983b)

$$PF_\infty = \frac{\alpha-1}{\alpha-1 + (2-\alpha)(\rho+\lambda_P) \int_0^\infty \psi(a) e^{-\rho a} da}$$

If loss of Q-cells is a Poisson process with rate λ_Q, then $\psi(a)=$ $=\exp(-\lambda_Q a)$ and hence

$$PF_\infty = \frac{\alpha-1}{\alpha-1 + (2-\alpha) \dfrac{\rho+\lambda_P}{\rho+\lambda_Q}} \qquad (6.20)$$

In the special case $\lambda_P = \lambda_Q$, this reduces to the well-known formula $PF_\infty = \alpha-1$ (see Sec.3).

7. The Kendall-Takahashi model

In Sec. 5 we derived formulae for the phase indices of asynchronously
growing cell populations, assuming uniform phase durations and cycle
time. Then we introduced a model with distributed cycle time and derived some general laws, but the phase indices were not considered in
detail. The next step will be to include distributed phase durations
into the analysis and to generalize the results of Sec. 5 concerning
the phases. Several mathematical models which are essentially equivalent have been proposed (see Sundareshan and Fundakowski, 1984, and
references there). The model which is discussed here makes it easy to
include various cytotoxic drug effects (see Chap. III).

If the length of each phase is a random variable as the cycle time is,
cells cannot be assigned to a certain phase according to their chronological age. Therefore the concept of functional age will be used in
this section. We assume that functional age is a discrete variable
that can take the integer values $1,2,...,n$. Then the cell cycle is divided into n stages or compartments. These stages are aggregated into
four groups according to the four phases. The passage from stage i to
stage i+1 ($i=1,...,n-1$) is a Poisson process with rate a_i, i.e. a random process, such that the probability of transition from i to i+1 in
a time interval of length Δt is $a_i \Delta t$. Cell loss at stage i is a Poisson
process with rate λ_i. Cells at stage n divide and the daughters pass
to stage 1, following the same law with rate a_n. Each cell behaves independently of every other with regard to passage times. The constants
a_i are called the passage rates.

These assumptions constitute the model that was first proposed by
Kendall (1948) and later adapted to cell kinetics by Takahashi (1966).

Kendall's stochastic treatment of the model considers the probabilities $p_{ik}(t)$ that k cells are at stage i at time t, and is important for the study of carcinogenesis and of small cell colonies in vitro. The simpler deterministic view adopted by Takahashi is justified, when the number of cells under study is large.

Following Takahashi we assume that at any time the actual number is equal to the expected or mean number of cells at stage i. Let $x_i(t)$ denote the number of cells at stage i at time t. The total number of P-cells is then

$$P(t) = \sum_{i=1}^{n} x_i(t)$$

With $n_i(t) = x_i(t)/P(t)$ (i=1,...,n) we form the vector $(n_1,...,n_n)$, which is called the age distribution of P-cells. It describes the distribution of cells among the various stages of functional age.

First we consider a special case of the model, with only four stages, each stage corresponding to a phase of the cycle (Fig. 8), and with $a_i=1$, $\lambda_i=0$, (i=1,...,4).

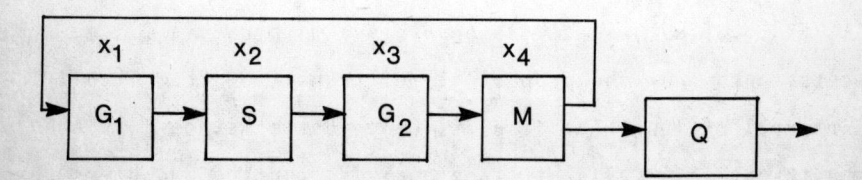

Fig.8: Special case of the Takahashi model with 4 stages.

The x_i satisfy the following system of differential equations (which will be derived later, when the general case is treated):

$$x_1' = \alpha x_4 - x_1$$
$$x_2' = x_1 - x_2$$
$$x_3' = x_2 - x_3 \tag{7.1}$$
$$x_4' = x_3 - x_4$$

Here and in the sequel, a prime denotes the derivative with respect to t.
If this system has a solution of the form $x_k = c_k e^{\lambda t} \neq 0$ (k=1,2,3,4),
then $x_k' = \lambda x_k$ and hence $(\lambda+1)x_k = x_{k-1}$ (k=2,3,4) and $(\lambda+1)x_1 = \alpha x_4$.
Therefore,

$$(\lambda+1)^4 x_4 = (\lambda+1)^3 x_3 = \ldots = \alpha x_4$$

i.e. $(\lambda+1)^4 = \alpha$ because $x_4 \neq 0$. Let ß be the positive real root of
the equation $z^4 = \alpha$ and put

$$\rho = \beta-1 \qquad (\beta = \sqrt[4]{\alpha} > 0)$$

The set of functions $x_k(t) = \beta^{4-k} e^{\rho t}$ (k=1,2,3,4) is a solution of the
system (1) with constant age distribution and exponential growth.

Now we establish the solution which corresponds to the subpopulation
of labelled cells after pulse labelling with H^3-Thymidine. For k=1,2,3,4
consider the functions

$$f_k(t) = e^{(\beta-1)t} + (-1)^k e^{-(\beta+1)t} - 2e^{-t}\cos(\beta t - k \frac{\pi}{2})$$
$$x_k(t) = \beta^{4-k} f_k(t) \tag{7.2}$$

which satisfy $f_k' = \beta f_{k-1} - f_k$ for k=2,3,4 and hence

$$x_k' = x_{k-1} - x_k \qquad (k=2,3,4)$$

The first equation of the system (1) is satisfied because $f_1' = \beta f_4 - f_1$ and $x_1' = \beta^3 f_1' = \beta^4 f_4 - \beta^3 f_1 = \alpha x_4 - x_1$. Furthermore, $x_2(0) = 4\beta^2$ and $x_k(0) = 0$ for k=1,3,4. This means that at t=0 all cells are in S-phase. The functions f_k exhibit heavily damped oscillations of period $2\pi/\beta$ and approach rapidly the functions $\beta^{4-k} e^{\rho t}$ belonging to the constant age distribution.

After this preliminary discussion of a special case, we begin with the rigorous study of the Takahashi model (Takahashi, 1968). In this model it is assumed that there is no interaction between cells and no correlation between passage times through consecutive phases and through the cycle of mother and daughter cell. Concerning the phases, this assumption is supported by experiments (Schultze et al., 1979, see Chap.II, Sec.7). The phase φ ($\varphi = G_1$, S, G_2, or M) is subdivided into n_φ stages, and the passage from any stage of phase φ to the next stage is a Poisson process with rate a_φ. Equally, cell loss from phase φ is a Poisson process with rate λ_φ. These assumptions imply that the duration of phase φ has the gamma distribution

$$\Gamma_\varphi(x) = c\frac{(cx)^{k-1}}{(k-1)!} \ e^{-cx} \qquad (c = a_\varphi + \lambda_\varphi, \ k = n_\varphi) \qquad (7.3)$$

The mean μ and variance σ^2 of this distribution can be expressed by k and c:

$$\mu = k/c \qquad\qquad \sigma^2 = k/c^2 \qquad\qquad (7.4a)$$

and vice versa:

$$c = \mu/\sigma^2 \qquad\qquad k = \mu^2/\sigma^2 \qquad\qquad (7.4b)$$

Since a single cell leaves stage i with probability $(a_i + \lambda_i)\Delta t$ and independently of other cells, the efflux out of stage i during time Δt is

$(a_i + \lambda_i) x_i \Delta t$ and the influx into stage i is $a_{i-1} x_{i-1} \Delta t$. In this deterministic view $(a_i + \lambda_i) \Delta t$ is the ratio of the number of cells leaving stage i and the number of cells present at stage i. The difference between influx and efflux yields the increment

$$x_i(t+\Delta t) - x_i(t) = \{a_{i-1} x_{i-1}(t) - (a_i + \lambda_i) x_i(t)\} \Delta t \quad (i=2,\ldots,n).$$

Since each cell leaving stage n produces in the mean α cells of stage 1, the term $a_{i-1} x_{i-1}$ is replaced by $\alpha a_n x_n$ when i=1. Division through Δt and $\Delta t \to 0$ yields the differential equations

$$x_1' = \alpha a_n x_n - (a_1 + \lambda_1) x_1$$

$$x_i' = a_{i-1} x_{i-1} - (a_i + \lambda_i) x_i \quad (i=2,3,\ldots,n) \tag{7.5}$$

It is suggested by the special case (1) that this system has a solution of the form $x_i(t) = \eta_i e^{\rho t}$ $(i=1,\ldots,n)$ where η_i is constant. Inserting in eq.(5) we get

$$\alpha a_n \eta_n - (a_1 + \lambda_1 + \rho) \eta_1 = 0$$

$$a_{i-1} \eta_{i-1} - (a_i + \lambda_i + \rho) \eta_i = 0 \quad (i=2,3,\ldots,n) \tag{7.6}$$

and therefore

$$\eta_n = \frac{a_{n-1}}{a_n + \lambda_n + \rho} \, \eta_{n-1}$$

$$= \frac{a_{n-1} \cdots a_1}{(a_n + \lambda_n + \rho) \cdots (a_2 + \lambda_2 + \rho)} \, \eta_1$$

$$= \frac{\alpha a_n \cdots a_1}{(a_n + \lambda_n + \rho) \cdots (a_1 + \lambda_1 + \rho)} \, \eta_n$$

Since $\eta_n \neq 0$, we obtain the "characteristic equation"

$$(1 + \frac{\rho+\lambda_1}{a_1})(1 + \frac{\rho+\lambda_2}{a_2}) \cdots (1 + \frac{\rho+\lambda_n}{a_n}) = \alpha \qquad (7.7)$$

which has always a unique real solution ρ. When eq.(7) has been solved for ρ, eq.(6) can be solved for the η_i. In the Appendix it is shown that any solution of the system (5) satisfies

$$\lim_{t \to \infty} x_i(t)e^{-\rho t} = c_o \eta_i \qquad (i=1,2,\ldots,n)$$

where c_o is a constant. The vector $(\eta_1, \eta_2, \ldots, \eta_n)$ that satisfies eq.(6) and $\eta_1 + \eta_2 + \cdots + \eta_n = 1$ is called the stable age distribution.

Now we consider the special case in which all passage rates and all loss rates are equal, say $a_i = b$, $\lambda_i = \lambda_p$ $(i=1,\ldots,n)$. Then eq.(7) is reduced to the simple form

$$(1 + \frac{\rho+\lambda_p}{b})^n = \alpha \qquad (7.8)$$

and hence

$$\rho = b(\sqrt[n]{\alpha} - 1) - \lambda_p \qquad (7.9)$$

The cycle time is distributed according to eq.(3) with $c = b + \lambda_p$, $k = n$, and its mean and variance are given by

$$\overline{T}_C = \frac{n}{b+\lambda_p} \qquad\qquad var(T_C) = \frac{n}{(b+\lambda_p)^2} \qquad (7.10)$$

The mean and variance of the duration of phase φ are expressed in the same way, with n_φ instead of n, and hence

$$\overline{T}_\varphi / \overline{T}_C = n_\varphi / n \qquad (7.11)$$

i.e. the mean duration of phase φ is proportional to the number of stages representing it.

With ρ taken from eq.(9), the i-th equation of the system (6) becomes

$$b\, n_{i-1} - b\, ^n\sqrt{\alpha}\; n_i = 0 \qquad (7.12)$$

Therefore, the stable age distribution is given by

$$n_i = \frac{q-1}{\alpha-1}\, q^{n-i} \qquad (i=1,\ldots,n)$$

where $q = {}^n\sqrt{\alpha}$ (see Fig.9).

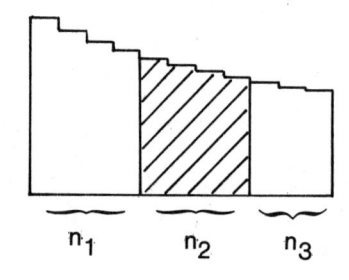

Fig.9: Stable age distribution in the Takahashi model

With this background, it is easy to derive the analogues of the formulae for the phase indices found in Sec. 5. Let n_1, n_2, n_3 be nonnegative integers and let $m = n_1+n_2+n_3 \leq n$. The fraction of cells in stages n_1+1 to n_1+n_2 (shaded area in Fig.9) with respect to all cells in stages 1 to m is

$$\frac{A}{B} = \frac{q^{n_3}(1+q+\ldots+q^{n_2-1})}{1+q+\ldots+q^{m-1}}$$

$$= q^{n_3}\; \frac{q^{n_2}-1}{q^m-1}$$

Remembering that $q = {}^n\sqrt{\alpha} = \exp(\frac{1}{n}\log\alpha)$, we get

$$\frac{A}{B} = e^{\log \alpha (n_3/n)} \{e^{\log \alpha (n_2/n)} - 1\}\{e^{\log \alpha (m/n)} - 1\}^{-1} \qquad (7.13)$$

and applying (5.9) to both terms in parantheses:

$$\frac{A}{B} \simeq \frac{n_2}{m} e^{1/2 \log \alpha (2n_3+n_2-m)/n} \qquad (7.13a)$$

$$= \frac{n_2}{m} e^{1/2 \log \alpha (n_3-n_1)/n}$$

In the special case m=n we obtain, when (5.9) is applied only to the first term in parantheses:

$$\frac{A}{B} = \frac{\log \alpha}{\alpha - 1} \frac{n_2}{n} e^{\log \alpha (1/2 \, n_2 + n_3)/n} \qquad (7.13b)$$

Let us apply these results to the phase indices. We assume that a phase φ with mean duration $\overline{T}_\varphi$ is represented by n_2 stages and that the last n_3 stages represent the phases after φ, which have mean duration $\overline{T}_3$. From eq.(11) we obtain

$$n_2/n = \overline{T}_\varphi/\overline{T}_C \qquad n_3/n = \overline{T}_3/\overline{T}_C \qquad (7.14)$$

Therefore, the only difference between (7.13), (7.13a) and their counterparts (5.8), (5.8a) is that ρ has been replaced by $\log \alpha/\overline{T}_C$, and phase durations (cycle times) by the mean.

Cell loss has not been considered in Sec. 5, but the generalization of the results to the case with age-independent cell loss is straightforward. Indeed, eq.(6.14) implies that the stable age distribution of a cell population with uniform cycle time and cell loss at a constant rate λ_p is $A_o \exp\{-(\rho+\lambda_p)a\}$, since $\varphi(a)=\exp(-\lambda_p a)$ in this case. Therefore, it is sufficient to replace ρ by $\rho+\lambda_p$ in eq.(5.8), (5.8a), and (5.8b).

Consequently, we are left with the problem of estimating the difference between $\rho+\lambda_P$ and $\log \alpha/\overline{T}_C$. From eq.(9) and (10) we obtain

$$\rho+\lambda_P-\log \alpha/\overline{T}_C = n(\sqrt[n]{\alpha} - 1 - \log \sqrt[n]{\alpha})/\overline{T}_C$$

Now we write $h = \sqrt[n]{\alpha} - 1$ and use the inequalities

$$0 < h - \log(1+h) < \frac{1}{2}h^2$$

which are due to a property of the alternating series

$$\log (1+h) = h - \frac{1}{2}h^2 + \frac{1}{3}h^3 - \dots,$$

and the inequality $e^x-1 < xe^x$ applied to $x = \log \alpha/n$. We obtain

$$0 < \sqrt[n]{\alpha} - 1 - \log \sqrt[n]{\alpha} < \frac{1}{2} (\sqrt[n]{\alpha} - 1)^2$$

$$< \frac{(\log \alpha)^2}{2n^2} \exp(\frac{2}{n} \log \alpha)$$

and consequently

$$0 < \frac{\rho+\lambda_P}{\log \alpha/T_C} - 1 < \frac{\log \alpha}{2n} \sqrt[n]{\alpha}^2$$

The last term is the relative error which is sufficiently small in most cases where the model is adapted to a real tumor. Indeed, the variance in cycle time observed in experimental animal tumors and in many human tumors suggests the use of $n \geq 10$ stages, and for $\alpha \leq 2$, $n \geq 10$ the error term is <0.04. Therefore, the formulae of Sec. 5 are good approximations in all cases in which the Takahashi model with equal passage rates can be applied.

II. DETERMINATION OF CELL KINETIC PARAMETERS

Cell kinetic experiments

Although the basic models of population growth apply to cells as well
as to animals and men, the methods used to determine kinetic parameters are quite different in the two areas. In demography and partly
in population biology the parameters (e.g. mean life span) are obtained by observations on a certain number of individuals at several stages
of their life or during their whole life. But it is impossible to pick
up any individual cell in vivo and perform subsequent observations on
it. This difficulty in the study of cells however is compensated for by
the possibility of observing at any given time a great number of cells
and of performing experiments. Observing a great number of cells allows
the determination of certain phase indices, and then the relative duration of these phases can be calculated with appropriate formulae. More
information is supplied by the observation of synchronous instead of
asynchronous cell populations. Synchronization can be achieved by special experimental techniques (see the survey by Nias and Fox, 1971)
or by selection of a synchronous subpopulation (e.g. by labelling cells
in S-phase). Since the phase indices of synchronous cell populations
are varying, samples of the population are taken and prepared for in-
spection at different times during the course of the experiment. If in
a study in vivo only one sample can be taken per animal, then the samples have to be taken at different times from different animals which
have received the same treatment. Each sample reflects the state of the
population at the time when it was taken, and thus it is possible to
draw curves of the observable quantities over time. In the analysis of
these curves mathematics are very helpful.

In the following sections the most important experimental techniques are reviewed, and it is shown how the data obtained can be used to calculate certain parameters. Each section (except 6 and 7) consists of three paragraphs: the first describes briefly how the experiment is run, the second predicts the result applying a certain model, and the third indicates model-based procedures for inferring kinetic parameters from experimental data. All methods of evaluation, except the analysis of FLM-curves, can be carried out with no more than a pocket calculator. Statistical aspects of the evaluation of cell kinetic data are not considered, but the interested reader may consult Amlacher (1974), Aherne (1977) or Staudte (1981). Equally, flow cytofluorometry has been omitted. The computational aspects of this technique are discussed thoroughly by Eisen (1977) and Zietz and Nicolini (1978). Experiments directed to measure the action of cytotoxic drugs are discussed in Chapter III.

Throughout this chapter, we assume a stable age distribution and exponential growth (including the special case of zero growth) at the beginning of the experiment. Unless a metaphase arrest technique is applied, the stable age distribution of the total cell population is supposed to be maintained during the experiment, although there may be subpopulations of synchronous cells. For the sake of simplicity, it is assumed that only Q-cells (sterile cells) are subject to loss. As indicated at the end of Chapter I, the analysis follows the same lines if loss of P-cells at a constant age-independent rate λ_p is admitted, but then the growth rate ρ cannot be estimated from labelling data because it appears always as $\rho + \lambda_p$. More specific assumptions are stated in each section.

1. Pulse labelling

a) Experiment

When a single dose of H^3-Thymidine is injected into an animal, a part
is incorporated into the DNA of cells in S-phase and the rest is quick-
ly (≤ 1 hour) broken down to nonutilizable products. At a time $\frac{1}{2}$ to 1
hour after injection, the animal is killed and a sample of the cell
population under study is taken. During the fixation procedure the non-
incorporated Thymidine and its derivatives are washed out. The same effect can be produced with cells in vitro, when they are exposed to H^3-
Thymidine during a short time, e.g. 30 minutes, and then washed.

After fixation, an autoradiograph is prepared, i.e. the specimen is
covered with a photographic emulsion, kept in complete darkness and at
low temperature during some days or weeks, and then developed. Those
cells which were synthesizing DNA during exposure to H^3-Thymidine will
have black silver grains deposited in the emulsion above them. Some
other cells may also have a few silver grains due to background noise.
For each cell the number of grains is recorded, and a distribution of
grain numbers with two peaks is obtained. Then a threshold number is
chosen (the grain number at the minimum between the peaks), and cells
are classified as labelled, if their grain number is greater than the
threshold, and unlabelled otherwise. The fraction of labelled cells is
called the labelling index (LI).

The activity of the H^3-Thymidine used must be so low, that the kinetics of the cells under study are not disturbed. The physical and biological problems of the labelling method are treated thoroughly by
Schultze (1969) and Amlacher (1974).

b) Theory

We define the point t=0 of the time scale to be the end of exposure to H^3-Thymidine. In vitro exposure can be stopped abruptly and hence this definition is clear. In vivo we may argue that the concentration declines to very low values within a certain time, say 30 minutes, and that the end of exposure occurs at 30 minutes after injection.

We assume that the cell population can be described by the Takahashi model with equal passage rates. This includes the following assumptions:

- the transit time through phase φ is gamma-distributed with mean μ_φ and variance σ_φ^2,

- transit times through consecutive phases are uncorrelated,

- the ratio $\mu_\varphi/\sigma_\varphi^2 = b$ is independent of the phase,

- the ratio $\mu_\varphi^2/\sigma_\varphi^2$ is an integer n_φ.

We denote the labelling index at time t with LI_t. With the preceding assumptions, an expression for LI_0 is readily obtained. For $t > 0$ we need additional assumptions to be stated later. Note that in the common terminology the term "labelling index" applies to LI_0 only.

LI_0 is the fraction of labelled cells at the end of exposure. What is the value of LI_0? All cells that were in S-phase during the whole exposure time are labelled. Some cells, which were reaching the border S/G_2 at the beginning of exposure, have completed DNA-synthesis without taking label (strictly speaking: the amount of label results in a grain number below the threshold). But this defect is roughly compensated for by some cells which entered S-phase during exposure and have taken-up enough label to produce a grain number above the threshold. Therefore LI_0 equals the S-phase index. Using eqs. (5.10) and (5.10a) from Chap.I we get

$$LI_0 = \frac{PF}{\alpha-1} e^{\rho T_3} (e^{\rho T_S}-1) \qquad (1.1a)$$

and

$$LI_0 = k_S \, PF \, \frac{T_S}{T_C} \qquad (1.1b)$$

where the correction factor k_S is given by

$$k_S = \exp\{ \tfrac{1}{2}\rho(T_{G_2M}-T_{G_1}) \}$$

Before considering LI_t for $t>0$ we should discuss the question whether the daughter cells of a labelled cell will always be recognized as labelled. For this end we look more in detail upon DNA-synthesis and mitosis. During DNA-synthesis the double strand of each chromosome is separated into single strands, and then a new complementary strand for each single strand is built. Hence, when this process is completed, each chromosome is composed of an old and a new strand, and in la-

belled cells only the new strand carries H^3-Thymidine. At the first division after labelling, each daughter cell gets a complete set of chromosomes of the mixed type (one strand labelled, one unlabelled). Hence,
in the first post-labelling generation the variation of the number of
grains per cell is small. But after completion of the next S-phase,
one half of the chromosomes are unlabelled and one half are of the mixed type. If the distribution of chromosomes among the parts of the dividing cell is random with respect to label, then the probability of
one daughter cell inheriting considerably less radioactivity than the
other increases with each division. Furthermore, the mean radioactivity per cell is halved after each cycle, and, therefore, the threshold number has to be adjusted in an appropriate way. But ultimately
the radioactivity in descendants of labelled cells decreases to a level too low for distinguishing them from descendants of unlabelled
cells.

Now let us consider LI_t for $0 < t \leq T_3 + T_C$ and assume that

    - phase durations are uniform

    - the life span of Q-cells is at least T_C.

Then, for $0 < t \leq T_3 = T_{G_2} + T_M$ the number of labelled cells does not increase, but the whole population is growing with rate ρ, hence

$$LI_t = e^{-\rho t} LI_0 \qquad\qquad (0 < t \leq T_3) \qquad\qquad (1.2a)$$

During the time between T_3 and $T_3 + T_S$ all labelled cells pass through
mitosis and the number of labelled cells increases by the factor 2,
provided that no labelled cells are lost, while the total number of

cells increases by the factor $e^{\rho T_S}$. Therefore

$$LI_{T_3+T_S} = 2 e^{-\rho(T_3+T_S)} LI_0 \qquad (1.2b)$$

For $T_3+T_S \leq t \leq T_3+T_C$ the number of labelled cells does not increase, so we have $LI_t = 2e^{-\rho t} LI_0$ and in particular, since $e^{\rho T_C} = \alpha$,

$$LI_{T_C} = \frac{2}{\alpha} LI_0 \qquad (1.2c)$$

The time course of LI_t is shown in Fig.1. The full line corresponds to the assumption of uniform phase durations, the dotted line gives the correction due to small variations of transit times.

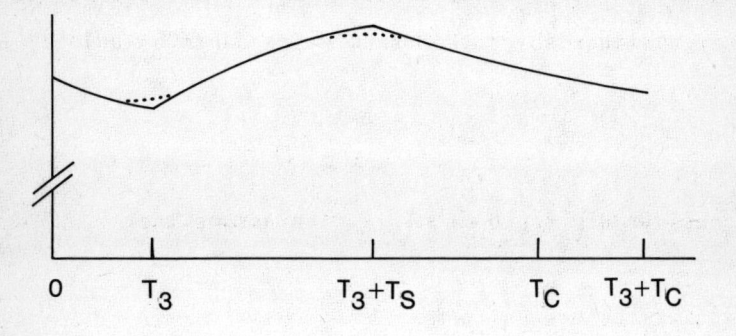

Fig.1: Fraction of labelled cells after pulse labelling

For $t > T_3+T_C$ it is difficult to give an accurate formula for LI_t, since the loss of labelled Q-cells can no longer be neglected. But if we disregard the difficulty of detecting scarcely labelled cells, then we can calculate the limit of LI_t for $t \to \infty$. We assume that

- the Takahashi model with equal passage rates applies,

- all descendants of labelled cells are labelled.

According to the last assumption, labelled cells follow the same kinetics as unlabelled cells, hence they approach a stable age distribution with growth fraction PF. Let t_∞ be the time when the stable age distribution is reached. Further, let P and N be the number of P-cells and the total number of cells, respectively; and let P* and N* be the numbers of the corresponding labelled subpopulations. Then

$$\frac{P^*(t_\infty)}{N^*(t_\infty)} = \frac{P(t_\infty)}{N(t_\infty)} = PF \tag{1.3}$$

and hence

$$LI_{t_\infty} = \frac{N^*(t_\infty)}{N(t_\infty)} = \frac{P^*(t_\infty)}{P(t_\infty)}$$

According to Theorem 3 of the Appendix this ratio is equal to T_S/T_C. Therefore

$$\frac{P^*(t_\infty)}{P(t_\infty)} = \frac{T_S}{T_C} \quad \text{and}$$

$$LI_{t_\infty} = \frac{T_S}{T_C} \tag{1.4}$$

From this and (1.1b) we get

$$PF = \frac{LI_0}{LI_{t_\infty}} k_S^{-1} \tag{1.5}$$

However, this method of determination of the growth fraction requires that t_∞ be less than the time at which labelled cells exhibit grain numbers near the background level. This condition is likely to be satisfied, if the life span of Q-cells does not exceed 3 or 4 cycle times, i.e. if unlabelled Q-cells die and are replaced by labelled Q- cells within that range of time.

c) Evaluation

If only LI_0 has been measured, no further evaluation is needed. If LI_{T_C} or LI_{t_∞} have been measured in addition, then (1.2c) resp. (1.5) may be used to obtain estimates of α resp. PF. The accuracy of these estimates depends on the mode and the rate of cell loss, as explained in paragraph b). If T_S/T_C is known from other experiments, PF can be obtained with (1.1b).

2. Continuous labelling

a) Experiment

A cell population is continuously exposed to H^3-Thymidine. In vivo this may be achieved by repeated injections. At different times samples are taken and autoradiographs prepared. For each sample the labelling index is determined as in pulse labelling. This index, which is always increasing with time, is called the index of continuous labelling (CL).

b) Theory

Let exposure begin at t=0. As an idealization we assume that cells initially in S-phase get the label immediately and that other cells are labelled at the moment when they enter the S-phase. We denote the index of continuous labelling at time t with CL_t.

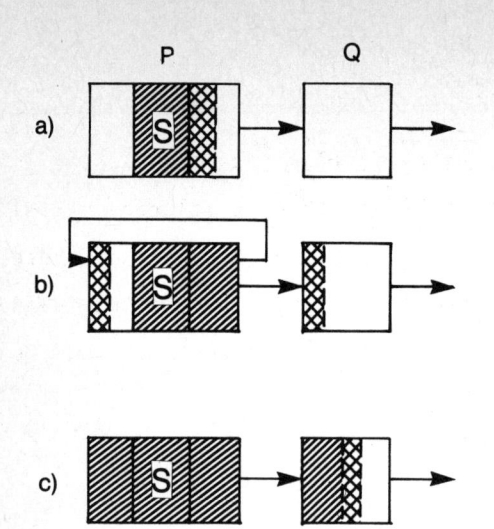

Fig.2: Continuous labelling
of a cell population in steady
state. Areas (recently) occupied
by labelled cells are (double)
shaded.

a: $0 \leq t \leq T_3$. Unlabelled cells
are replaced by labelled cells
in P. No labelled cells in Q.

b: $T_3 \leq t \leq T_3 + T_1$. Unlabelled
cells are replaced by labelled
cells in P and Q.

c: $T_3 + T_1 \leq t$. Unlabelled cells
are replaced by labelled cells
in Q.

The steady state ($\rho = 0$) and the case $\rho > 0$ must be treated separately.
For the steady state we assume

- uniform phase durations

- uniform life span T_Q of Q-cells.

Then PF $= T_C/(T_C + T_Q)$, since in a steady state system the number of
cells in a given compartment is proportional to the passage time (see
Sec.1, Chap. I). Between time 0 and T_3, unlabelled cells in G_2 and
M are replaced by labelled cells and CL_t increases linearly from
$PF(T_S/T_C)$ to $PF(T_S+T_3)/T_C$. Graphically this gives a straight line with
slope PF/T_C, which intersects the time axis at $t = -T_S$ (Fig.3). Between
time T_3 and $T_3 + T_1$ the increase of CL_t is accelerated, because division of labelled cells has begun and labelling of unlabelled cells
at the G_1/S boundary is continued. The value PF is reached at t =
$= T_3 + \frac{1}{2}T_1$.

At $t = T_3 + T_1$ all P-cells are labelled, but CL_t continues to increase, until all Q-cells are labelled at $t=T_3+T_Q$ (Fig.3).

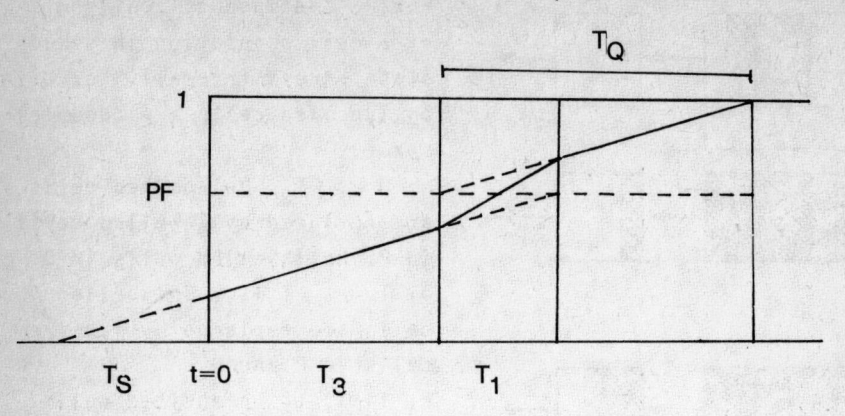

Fig.3: Index of continuous labelling in a steady state cell population

For the case $\rho > 0$ we assume

- uniform phase durations

- loss of Q-cells at a constant rate λ.

Again we have a slow increase of CL_t for $0 \leq t \leq T_3$ and $t > T_3+T_1$ and an accelerated increase for $T_3 \leq t \leq T_3+T_1$. At time $t \leq T_3$ all cells with age between T_1 and T_1+T_S+t are labelled (Fig.4). Therefore the fraction of labelled cells at time t is obtained from (5.8, Chap. I) where τ_2 is to be replaced by T_S+t and τ_3 by T_3-t:

$$CL_t = \frac{PF}{\alpha-1} \, e^{\rho(T_3-t)} \{ e^{\rho(T_S+t)} -1 \} \qquad (2.1)$$

If we apply (5.8a, Chap. I) with $\tau_1=T_1$, $\tau_2=T_S+t$, $\tau_3=T_3-t$, then

$$CL_t = PF \, \frac{T_S+t}{T_C} \, e^{\frac{1}{2}\rho(T_3-t-T_1)} \qquad (2.2)$$

and, provided that T_3 is near T_1,

$$CL_t = PF \frac{T_S+t}{T_C} e^{-\frac{1}{2}\rho t} \tag{2.2a}$$

Eqs. (1) and (2) may be used alternatively.

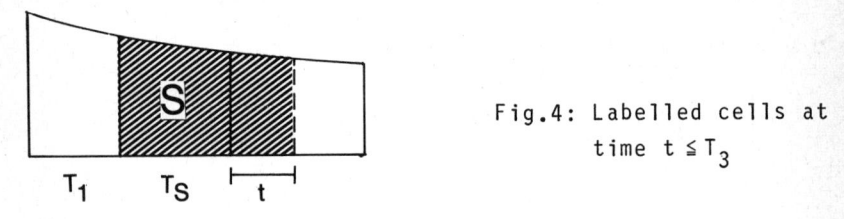

Fig.4: Labelled cells at time $t \leq T_3$

For $T_3 \leq t \leq T_3+T_1$ the term $1-e^{\rho(T_3-t)}$ has to be added, but we omit the proof of this fact because we will not use it.

Now we consider $t \geq T_3+T_1$. The assumption of uniform phase durations implies that at $t=T_3+T_1$ all P-cells are labelled. Let N be the number of all cells and Q_u the number of unlabelled Q-cells. Then the fraction of unlabelled cells is

$$1-CL_t = Q_u/N \qquad (t \geq T_1+T_3)$$

Since no unlabelled Q-cells are produced for $t \geq T_1+T_3$, the time derivatives satisfy the equations

$$dQ_u/dt = -\lambda Q_u \qquad dN/dt = \rho N$$

and hence, applying the quotient rule of calculus, we obtain

$$\frac{d}{dt}(1-CL_t) = -(\rho+\lambda)\frac{Q_u}{N} = -(\rho+\lambda)(1-CL_t)$$

and, after integration,

$$1-CL_t = c e^{-(\rho+\lambda)t} \qquad (t \geq T_1+T_3) \tag{2.3}$$

Here, c is a constant of integration.

c) Evaluation

From the first part $(0 \leq t \leq T_3)$ of the CL-curve an estimate of T_S is obtained. In the steady state case this is evident from Fig.3. In the case of exponential growth eq. (1) has been used most frequently, assuming $PF = \alpha-1$ and neglecting the factor $e^{\rho(T_3-t)}$. This implies

$$\log(1+CL_t) = \rho T_S + \rho t \qquad (2.4)$$

If the values of this function are calculated from measured values of CL_t and plotted over the time axis, a straight line can be fitted to the points, which has slope ρ and intersects the time axis at $t=-T_S$ (Fig.5).

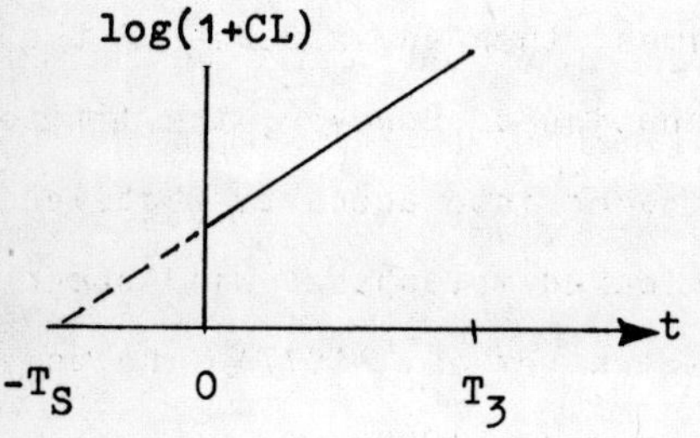

Fig.5: Graphical evaluation of continuous labelling experiment in the case $\rho > 0$.

A more accurate method of evaluation is based on eq. (2) or (2a). If ρ is known, a plot of $CL_t \exp(1/2\rho t)$ over time gives a straight line which has slope PF/T_C (see eq. (2a)) and intersects the time axis at $t=-T_S$.

The loss rate of Q-cells can be obtained from the third part of the CL-curve, if ρ is known. Indeed, eq. (3) implies

$$\log(1-CL_t) = \log c - (\rho+\lambda)t \qquad (t \geq T_1+T_3)$$

Therefore, if values of $\log(1-CL_t)$ for $t \geq T_1+T_3$ are plotted over time and a straight line is fitted, the slope of this line is $-(\rho+\lambda)$.

3. Metaphase arrest

Mitosis is the only phase of the cell cycle that is visible with the light microscope. The whole process and its different stages (prophase, metaphase, anaphase, telophase) have been described with much detail. Therefore it is easy to determine the mitotic index (I_M) at any moment, when a sample of cells is available.

a) Experiment

Cells are exposed to an agent, e.g. colchicine or colcemide, that arrests the cell cycle in the metaphase stage of mitosis by disturbing the formation of the metaphase spindle. When samples of the cell population are taken at different times, then an increase of the I_M is observed so long as exposure is continued. However, the limited life span of arrested cells must be taken into account. Whatever blocking agent is used, degeneration of blocked metaphases will occur if exposure is longer than 5-6 hours (Aherne et al., 1977). The dose has to be carefully chosen (Wright and Appleton, 1980).

b) Theory

We assume that
- all metaphases are arrested during the exposure period,
- arrested metaphases maintain their morphology during the exposure period,
- the agent doesn't kill or block cells in the phases G_1, S and G_2,
- cell death is absent or the chance to die is equal for sterile, resting and proliferating cells and for all phases,
- no resting cells enter the cycle,
- the cycle time is uniform.

The assumption on cell death implies that during the experiment, PF
is constant and equal to $\alpha-1$ (see p. 11), and is necessary, because
a preferential loss of Q-cells would cause an increase of PF, when
cell production is stopped.

Since the point at which cells are arrested (metaphase) is not at the
end of mitosis, the description of the initial phase of the experiment is somewhat complicated. Let t_1 be the time between metaphase
and the end of mitosis. After time t_1 the cohort of cells B (Fig.6)
has left mitosis and divided, and the cohort A has entered mitosis.
Cohort A is slightly greater than cohort B, but the whole population
size has increased, and therefore the I_M has remained constant. This
is valid for steady state populations ($\rho=0$) and for growing populations ($\rho>0$) as well.

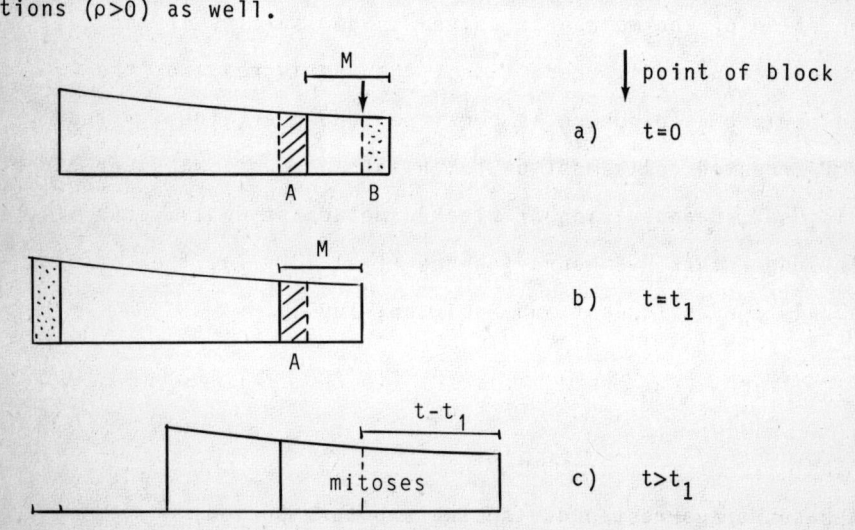

Fig.6: Metaphase arrest and flow of cells into mitosis

The further development has to consider the cases $\rho=0$ and $\rho>0$ separately. In the case $\rho=0$ (steady state) there is a constant flow of cells into mitosis and hence a linear increase of I_M from $(T_M/T_C)PF$ to PF, i.e.

$$I_M = PF \frac{t+(T_M-t_1)}{T_C} \qquad \text{for} \qquad t_1 \le t \le T_C-(T_M-t_1)$$

However, it should be noted that in steady state cell populations there is considerable loss of Q-cells, and hence our assumption on cell death is not valid. Therefore it is likely that in real situations the straight line in Fig.7 must be replaced by a curve with increasing slope.

In the case $\rho>0$ we argue as follows. The age distribution is shifted in the direction of increasing age, while the line separating mitotic from premitotic cells is fixed (Fig.6c). The part of the area to the right of this line represents the mitoses. Hence, applying (5.13, Chap.I) with $\tau_2=t+T_M-t_1$ and $\tau_3=0$ we get

$$I_M(t) = \frac{PF}{\alpha-1} \{\exp \rho(t+T_M-t_1)-1\}$$

Now, the assumption on cell loss implies PF $= \alpha-1$, and therefore

$$\log(1+I_M(t)) = \rho(t+T_M-t_1)$$

so long as $t \le T_C-(T_M-t_1)$. Later, when all P-cells have entered mitosis, I_M becomes constant.

c) Evaluation

In the case $\rho=0$ the observed values of I_M are plotted over the time axis, beginning at $t=t_1$, and a straight line is fitted to the points. The slope of this line is PF/T_C and the intercept (the distance between $t=t_1$ and the intersection with the time axis) is T_M (Fig.7, left).

In the case $\rho > 0$ the observed values of the "collection function" $\log(1+I_M)$ are plotted in the same way, and again a straight line is fitted to the points. The slope of this line is ρ and the intercept is T_M (Fig.7, right). If the experiment is continued long enough and if no degeneration of arrested cells occurs, then there is a point $(t = T_C - T_M + t_1)$, where the line with slope ρ becomes a parallel to the time axis with distance $\log(1+PF) = \log \alpha$.

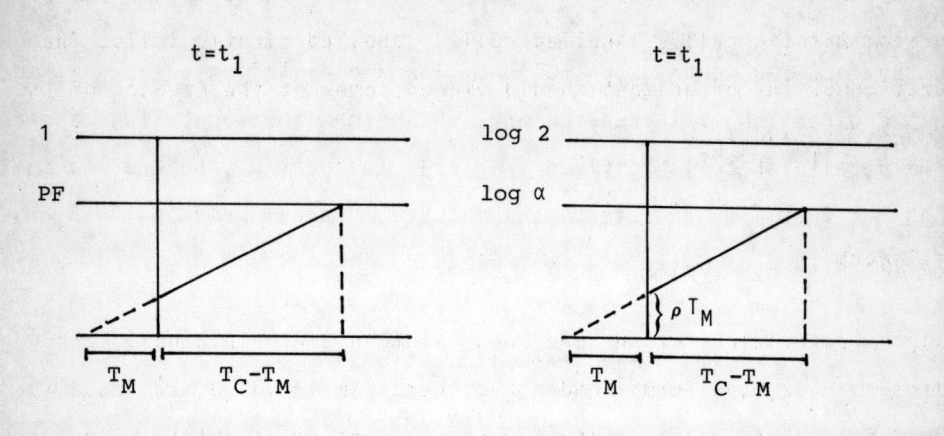

Fig.7: Evaluation of metaphase arrest
      Left: Steady state, I_M is plotted
      Right: Growing, $\log(1+I_M)$ is plotted

Thus, under favorable conditions, the parameters ρ, T_M, T_C and PF can be determined by this experiment. But if T_C is much longer than the life span of arrested cells, correct values of T_C and PF cannot be expected. This problem is overcome by an experiment, in which metaphase arrest and labelling are combined.

4. Continuous labelling with metaphase arrest

a) Experiment

Cells are exposed continuously to H^3-Thymidine and an agent blocking the cell cycle in mitosis. Samples are taken at different times, autoradiographs are prepared, and counts of three subpopulations are performed: mitotic cells, labelled cells, labelled mitotic cells. The duration of the experiment should exceed somewhat the greater of the numbers T_{G_1} and T_{G_2}.

b) Theory

All the assumptions of the preceding section are maintained. For the mitotic index, the formulae derived there remain valid. In Fig.8 the area of labelled cells is limited at the left by a vertical line, which moves from the G_1/S border to the left. Therefore we apply (5.8, Chap.I) with $\tau_2 = t+T_S$, $\tau_3 = T_{G_2}+T_M$. With $PF = \alpha-1$ we obtain

$$CL_t = e^{\rho T_3}\{e^{\rho(t+T_S)}-1\} \tag{4.1}$$

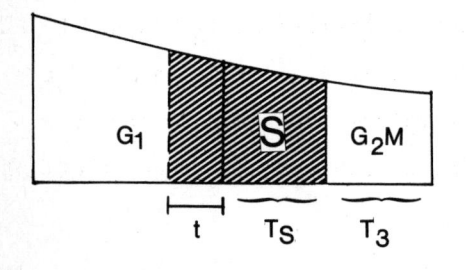

Fig.8: Labelled cells at time $t \leq T_{G_1}$ during mitotic block

This is valid for $0 \leq t \leq T_{G_1}$. At $t=T_{G_1}$ the plateau value

$$e^{\rho T_3}\{e^{\rho(T_{G_1}+T_S)}-1\} = e^{\rho T_C} - e^{\rho T_3}$$

is reached, because only cells initially in S or G_1 can be labelled.

Let T^* be the greater of the numbers T_{G_1} and T_{G_2}. At $t=T^*$ all P-cells are labelled or in mitosis, and no Q-cell is labelled. Hence the fraction of cells that are labelled or mitotic in $t=T^*$ is PF. This fraction cannot increase further, since no unlabelled cells enter mitosis or S-phase after $t=T^*$. It begins to decrease, when metaphases begin to degenerate. A correct estimate of PF is obtained, if metaphases are stable at least during time T^*.

c) Evaluation

This experiment can provide values of ρ, T_M, T_{G_1}, T_S, T_{G_2} and PF.

At first ρ and T_M are obtained as in the preceding section. Then autoradiographs are evaluated. The moment when the first labelled mitoses appear, is T_{G_2}. From (4.1) we get

$$1 + CL_t \ e^{-\rho T_3} = e^{\rho(t+T_S)}$$

where $T_3 = T_{G_2} + T_M$. Now the values of the function $\log(1 + CL_t \ e^{-\rho T_3})$, which is the analogue of the "collection function" of metaphase arrest, can be calculated from the observed values of CL_t and plotted over the time axis. A straight line can be fitted to these points, which crosses the time axis at $-T_S$. The plateau value of CL_t is reached at $t = T_{G_1}$.

In order to obtain PF, the fraction of cells that are labelled or mitotic, is plotted over time. The maximum or plateau value is PF.

5. Fractions of labelled mitoses (FLM)

a) Experiment

The method of fractions of labelled mitoses is based on pulse labelling with H^3-Thymidine (see Sec.1). At least 15 samples have to be
taken at different times after labelling throughout the presumed
length of the cycle. Autoradiographs are prepared and counts of the
number of mitoses and of labelled mitoses performed. After the first
peak of labelled mitoses the threshold number has to be reduced (or
exposure time of autoradiograph increased), because the amount of radioactivity per cell is halved during mitosis. A curve of fractions
of labelled mitoses (= number of labelled mitoses/number of all mitoses) over time is obtained.

b) Theory

In an introductory sense we first deduce the shape of the FLM curve
assuming uniform phase durations and $\alpha = 1$ (steady state).
We use a graphical representation in a plane, where the axes are time
and age and where the progress through the cycle of each cell is represented by a line with slope 1, which begins at t=0 or a=0 and ends
at $a=T_C$. The cohort of labelled cells is represented by the shaded
stripes (Fig.9). Labelled mitoses are double shaded.

Since the slope of the diagonal lines is 1, the length of G_1, S, G_2,
M marked on the vertical line t=0 is reproduced on the horizontal lines

$a=T_C-T_M$ and $a=T_C$. This leads immediately to the construction of the FLM curve in the upper part of Fig.9.

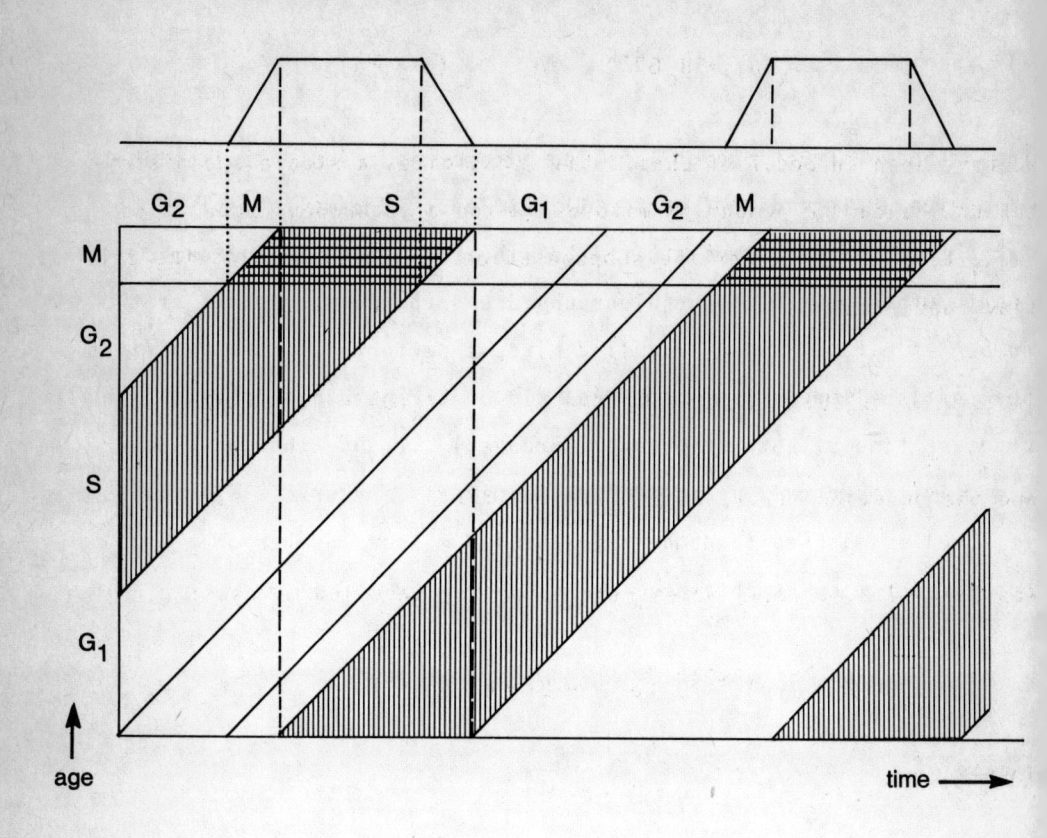

Fig.9: Construction of the ideal FLM curve

Now we adopt the general assumptions of the Takahashi model, i.e. we assume essentially

- gamma-distributed phase durations

- no correlation between successive phases.

Since the FLM does not depend on the behavior of Q-cells, we need no assumption concerning that. For the special case, in which each phase is represented by only one compartment and all passage rates a_i are 1, the FLM function is calculated easily. Suppose that for k=1,...,4 the number of cells in compartment k at time 0 is

$$x_k(0) = N_o \beta^{4-k} \qquad\qquad (\beta = \sqrt[4]{\alpha})$$

We have seen in Sec.7 of Chap.I that this gives a stable age distribution. Hence the number of mitoses in the asynchronous population is $x_4(t)=N_o e^{(\beta-1)t}$. For the subpopulation of labelled cells the initial conditions

$$x_2^*(0) = x_2(0) = N_o\beta^2 \qquad\qquad x_k^*(0) = 0 \qquad (k\neq 2)$$

and the equations (7.1, Chap.I) are valid.

Applying (7.2, Chap.I) we get the number of labelled mitoses:

$$x_4^*(t) = \frac{N_o}{4}\{e^{(\beta-1)t} - 2e^{-t}\cos\beta t + e^{-(1+\beta)t}\}$$

Therefore

$$FLM_t = \frac{x_4^*(t)}{x_4(t)} = \frac{1}{4}\{1 - 2e^{-\beta t}\cos\beta t + e^{-2\beta t}\}$$

This function is represented in Fig.10a. It corresponds to a cell population with extremely large variation of phase durations. The FLM curve of a cell population with small variation of phases is given in Fig.10b. It shows a sequence of waves with decreasing amplitude. An important fact is that the areas under the first and the second wave (and the following waves, if they are well separated) are equal. The proof of this follows.

The first (second) wave is produced by cells of the first (second) generation. Let x_k and y_k be the number of labelled cells of the first, respectively second generation in compartment k.

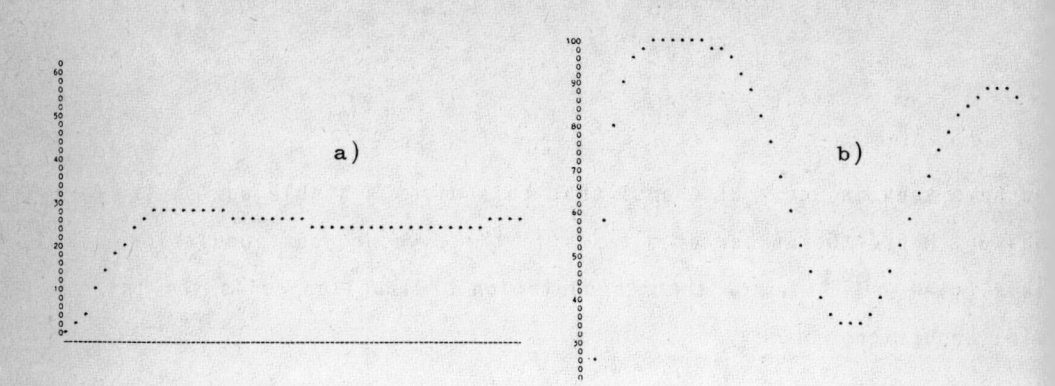

Fig.10: Fractions-of-labelled-mitoses curves calculated with a
computer program according to the Takahashi model

In an asynchronous cell population the number of mitoses at time t
is given by $m_0 e^{\rho t}$, where m_0 is the number of mitoses at time 0. Therefore the first and second wave of the FLM curve correspond to the
function

$$\frac{1}{m_0} e^{-\rho t} \cdot \sum_k x_k(t) \qquad \text{resp.} \qquad \frac{1}{m_0} e^{-\rho t} \sum_k y_k(t)$$

where the sum is taken over the compartments belonging to mitosis.
Therefore it is sufficient to show that for $k \in M$

$$\int_0^\infty x_k(t) e^{-\rho t} dt = \int_0^\infty y_k(t) e^{-\rho t} dt \qquad (5.1)$$

We will prove this relation for $k=n$. The case $k < n$ can be treated
in the same way.

The set of functions $x_1,\ldots,x_n$ satisfies eq. (7.5) of Chap.I with the
exception that $x_1' = -(a_1 + \lambda_1)x_1$. The y_k $(k=1,\ldots,n)$ satisfy the same

equations, but

$$y_1' = \alpha a_n x_n - (a_1 + \lambda_1) y_1$$

If we define $\xi_n = e^{-\rho t} x_n$ and $\eta_k = e^{-\rho t} y_k$ and write $b_i = a_i + \lambda_i$, then we obtain the following differential equations:

$$\eta_1' = \alpha a_n \xi_n - (b_1 + \rho) \eta_1$$

$$\eta_2' = a_1 \eta_1 - (b_2 + \rho) \eta_2$$

$$\vdots$$

$$\eta_{n-1}' = a_{n-2} \eta_{n-2} - (b_{n-1} + \rho) \eta_{n-1}$$

$$\eta_n' = a_{n-1} \eta_{n-1} - (b_n + \rho) \eta_n$$

Since cells of the second generation do not exist at t=0 and t=∞, we have $\int_0^\infty \eta_k'(t) dt = 0$ and therefore

$$(b_k + \rho) \int_0^\infty \eta_k(t) dt = a_{k-1} \int_0^\infty \eta_{k-1}(t) dt \qquad k = 2, \ldots, n$$

$$(b_1 + \rho) \int_0^\infty \eta_1(t) dt = \alpha a_n \int_0^\infty \xi_n(t) dt$$

Applying these relations successively, we get

$$\int_0^\infty \eta_n(t) dt = \frac{\alpha \cdot a_n \cdot a_{n-1} \cdots a_1}{(b_n + \rho)(b_{n-1} + \rho) \ldots (b_1 + \rho)} \int_0^\infty \xi_n(t) dt$$

But the ratio on the right side is 1, since ρ is a solution of the characteristic equation (7.7) from Chap.I. Thus, eq. (1) and the equality of the areas under the first and second wave is proved.

The subpopulation of labelled cells, which is synchronous at t=0, tends
to the stable age distribution according to the general law of decay
of synchrony. In the stable age distribution, there is a fixed ratio
between the number of mitoses M(t) and the number of all P-cells P(t).
Let t_∞ be the time, when the waves of the FLM curve have damped out,
i.e. when the labelled cells have reached the stable age distribution.
Then

$$\frac{M^*(t_\infty)}{P^*(t_\infty)} = \frac{M(t_\infty)}{P(t_\infty)}$$

and hence, applying (1.4), we get

$$\frac{M^*(t_\infty)}{M(t_\infty)} = \frac{P^*(t_\infty)}{P(t_\infty)} = \frac{T_S}{T_C} \tag{5.2}$$

This means that the FLM curve approaches ultimately the constant value
T_S/T_C.

c) Evaluation

Many computer programs for the analysis of FLM-curves have been developed (Hartmann et al. 1975). Evaluation of FLM-curves by hand is sat-
isfactory only if the first peak is high and the second peak well
pronounced. According to the "50% rule", the width of the first wave
at the 50% level gives T_S. This is exact in the case of the ideal FLM
curve in Fig.9, but when the first peak is far below 100%, it is wrong.
The distance between the first and the second ascent, which gives T_C,
cannot be assessed well if the second ascent is not steep. Nevertheless, in the case of rapid decay of synchrony, the final level of the

FLM, which is equal to T_S/T_C, is reached within a time covered by the experiment, and thus T_C is obtained if T_S has been determined from the first wave or from another experiment.

If the area under the second peak (if it is well pronounced) is less than the area under the first peak, caution is required. It may be that the threshold number is too high for labelled mitoses of the second generation, with lower grain count, to be recognized.

6. Double labelling

One of the most serious limitations of the FLM-method is the small mitotic index of many populations. The evaluation of autoradiographs becomes tedious, if thousands of cells have to be checked before a dozen mitoses are found. Therefore, double labelling techniques, which allow the generation of two or more differently-labelled subpopulations, are sometimes preferred. The "method of labelled S-phases" (Korr et al. 1983) is suited for the determination of the cycle time. If one is mainly interested in the duration of S-phase, then the following experiments should be considered.

a) Experiment 1: Double labelling with H^3

Pulse labelling is applied twice with equal activity at an interval shorter than S. Thus some cells are labelled twice. A sample is taken immediately after the second pulse and an autoradiograph is prepared. Unlabelled, weakly labelled, and strongly labelled cells are counted.

aa) Experiment 2: Double labelling with C^{14} and H^3

The cell population is first labelled with a pulse of C^{14}-Thymidine and then, after an interval Δt, with a pulse of H^3-Thymidine. A sample is taken immediately after the H^3-pulse and an autoradiograph with two layers of emulsion is prepared. The upper layer is penetrated only by ß-particles emitted by C^{14}, because they have a longer range than those emitted by H^3. With appropriate focusing of the microscope, silver grains in either of the layers become visible. Nuclei with grains only in the lower layer are purely H^3-labelled. Nuclei with grains in both layers may be C^{14}- and H^3-labelled or purely C^{14}-labelled, because some ß-particles emitted by C^{14} crash within the lower layer. But if the specific activity of the H^3-Thymidine is considerably higher than that of the C^{14}-Thymidine, purely C^{14}-labelled nuclei have only few grains in the lower layer and can be distinguished from double labelled nuclei (Schultze et al., 1976). Some authors report that they could distinguish two labelling classes only (Harris and Hoelzer, 1971). If this happens, then the experiment should be repeated with the reverse order of C^{14} and H^3. Then an accurate evaluation of the data is still possible, as will be shown in paragraph c).

b) Theory (H^3 twice)

We consider first double labelling with equal doses of H^3 and assume uniform phase durations. Cells may be lost at an age-independent rate from P and in any way from Q. Let Δt be the interval between pulses and look at Fig.11. When the second pulse starts, the cohort of cells

labelled by the first pulse is between the dotted lines. Cells within
the narrow bands W_1 and W_2 of width Δt become weakly labelled, and
cells between the bands become strongly labelled.

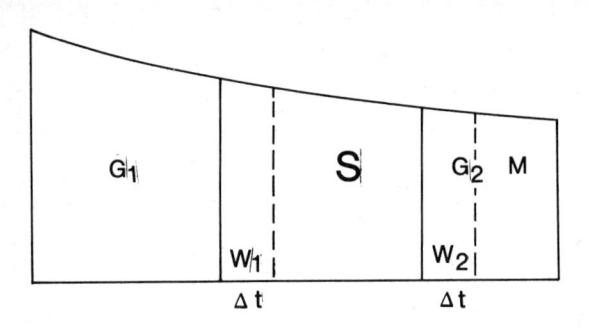

Fig.11: Position of differently labelled subpopulations in the
cell cycle

Let LI be the fraction of all labelled cells and LI_{st} (LI_w) the fraction of strongly (weakly) labelled cells. If the area $S-W_1$ is called
A and $S+W_2$ is called B, then applying (5.8a, Chap.I) with $\tau_1=\tau_3=\Delta t$,
$\tau_2=T_S-\Delta t$ we get

$$\frac{LI_{st}}{LI} = \frac{A}{B} = \frac{T_S-\Delta t}{T_S+\Delta t}$$

and consequently

$$T_S = \frac{LI + LI_{st}}{LI - LI_{st}} \Delta t \qquad (6.1)$$

It can be shown that eq. (1) is a good approximation for the case of
gamma-distributed phase durations, too. We omit the proof because double labelling with H^3 is much less used than other methods. It may
be that the difference in grain number of weakly and strongly labelled
cells in Experiment 1 is smaller than the variation of grain number
of equally labelled cells. Therefore a modification of the experiment

is proposed, where the activity in the 2nd dose is 10 times greater than in the 1st dose (Maurer-Schultze, personal communication). Then, nuclei labelled both times or only by the second pulse appear as strongly labelled, while nuclei labelled only by the 1st pulse are weakly labelled (the band W_2 in Fig.11). But the weakly labelled cells may be confounded with unlabelled cells, and so the problem of discrimination has only been transferred.

bb) Theory (C^{14} and H^3)

For the case of double labelling with C^{14} and H^3 we define the following labelling indices:

LI_{H^3} fraction of all H^3-labelled cells

$LI_{C^{14}}$ fraction of all C^{14}-labelled cells

$LI_{H^3\text{pure}}$ fraction of cells labelled only with H^3

$LI_{C^{14}\text{pure}}$ fraction of cells labelled only with C^{14}

These four fractions are not independent, since $LI_{C^{14}} + LI_{H^3\text{pure}} = LI_{H^3} + LI_{C^{14}\text{pure}}$. Various formulae which express ρ and T_S in terms of the different LI's have been derived assuming uniform phase durations (Knolle, 1984b). Now we show that the same formulae can be applied to cell populations which are described by the Takahashi model with equal passage rates. Accordingly, concerning the phases, we adopt the assumptions of Sec.1 (see p. 49). Cells may be lost in any way, but only from Q.

Remember that in this model each phase φ is represented by n_φ stages, that the probability of a cell to pass to the next stage in $(t, t+dt)$ is bdt and that the mean transit time through φ is $T_\varphi = n_\varphi/b$. The stable age distribution is given by a geometric series with factor $q = \sqrt[n]{\alpha}$ where n is the sum of the four integers n_φ (see Fig.9, Chap.I).

Now we write $n_3 = n_M + n_{G_2}$ and $n_2 = n_S$, and suppose that at $t=0$ there are z_o cells in the stage n of the cell cycle. Then the number of cells in S at time t is

$$z_S(t) = z_o e^{\rho t} q^{n_3}(1 + q + \ldots + q^{n_2 - 1}).$$

Furthermore, the number of cells entering S in $(t, t+dt)$ is $b z_o q^{n_2 + n_3} e^{\rho t} dt$, since b is the passage rate and $z_o q^{n_2 + n_3} e^{\rho t}$ is the number of cells at the stage immediately preceding S.

If pulse labelling with C^{14} occurs at $t=0$, then $z_S(0)$ cells become labelled with C^{14}. Those cells that enter S between $t=0$ and $t=\Delta t$ (the moment of H^3-labelling) become purely H^3-labelled. Their number is

$$z_{\Delta t} = b z_o q^{n_3 + n_2} \int_0^{\Delta t} e^{\rho s} ds,$$

and the integral can be approximated by $\Delta t \exp(\frac{1}{2}\rho\Delta t)$. Therefore

$$\frac{LI_{C^{14}}}{LI_{H^3 \text{pure}}} = \frac{1 + q + \ldots + q^{n_2 - 1}}{(\Delta t) b q^{n_2} \exp(\frac{1}{2}\rho\Delta t)}$$

Now we use the approximation

$$1+q+ \ldots +q^m \simeq (m+1)q^{m/2} \tag{6.2}$$

which follows from (5.9, Chap.I) on inserting $x=(m+1)\log q$ and $x=\log q$. (Since $x \leq \log 2$ the relative error is less than 0.02). If we write $v_1 = LI_{C14} : LI_{H^3 pure}$ and remember that $T_S = n_2/b$ (see eq. 7.10, 7.11, Chap.I), then we obtain

$$v_1 = \frac{T_S}{\Delta t} q^{-(n_2+1)/2} e^{-\rho \Delta t/2} \tag{6.3a}$$

Here, and in the rest of this section, T_S and T_C denote the mean of the S-phase and the cycle, respectively. At the end of Chap.I we have shown that ρ is greater than and close to $\log \alpha / T_C$. Furthermore, $q = \sqrt[n]{\alpha} \leq \sqrt[n]{2}$ is only slightly greater than 1. Therefore we obtain, using $q = \exp(\log \alpha / n)$ and (7.14, Chap.I),

$$q^{-(n_2+1)/2} = \exp \{ -\frac{n_2+1}{2n} \log \alpha \}$$

$$= \exp \{ -\frac{1}{2} (\frac{\log \alpha}{T_C} T_S + \frac{1}{n} \log \alpha) \}$$

$$\simeq \exp (-\frac{1}{2} \rho T_S).$$

Now eq. (3a) yields

$$T_S = v_1 \Delta t \exp \{ \frac{1}{2} \rho (T_S + \Delta t) \} \tag{6.4}$$

A formula for ρ is obtained in the following way.
All cells that are in S at $t = \Delta t$ become H^3-labelled. Therefore

$$LI_{H^3} = e^{\rho \Delta t} z_S(0) = e^{\rho \Delta t} LI_{C14}$$

and hence

$$\rho\Delta t = \log(LI_{H^3}) - \log(LI_{C^{14}}) \qquad (6.5)$$

But it may be that technical difficulties do not allow the determination of LI_{H^3} and that ρ is still unknown. Then a second double-labelling experiment, with C^{14} after H^3, should be performed. Doing so, cells that leave S between $t=0$ and $t=\Delta t$ become purely H^3-labelled, and cells that are in S at $t=\Delta t$ become C^{14}-labelled. Therefore, calculating the respective cell numbers and dividing, we obtain

$$\frac{LI_{C^{14}}}{LI_{H^3 pure}} = \frac{(1+q+ \ldots +q^{n_2-1})\exp(\rho\Delta t)}{(\Delta t)b\exp(\frac{1}{2}\rho\Delta t)}$$

$$\simeq \frac{n_2}{b\Delta t} q^{\frac{1}{2}(n_2-1)} e^{\frac{1}{2}\rho\Delta t}$$

If we denote the ratio $LI_{C^{14}} : LI_{H^3 pure}$ from this experiment with v_2, then

$$v_2 = \frac{T_S}{\Delta t} q^{(n_2-1)/2} e^{\rho\Delta t/2} \qquad (6.3b)$$

c) Evaluation
—————

Since eq. (1) gives an explicit expression for T_S, we pass immediately to eq. (4) and (3a/b). The calculation of ρ from eq. (5) is straightforward.

If ρ and v_1 are known, T_S can be calculated from eq. (3) by iteration, starting e.g. with $T_S=\Delta t$. There are two mathematical solutions, but it can be proved that the iteration process converges to the biological meaningful solution (Knolle, 1984b).

A simple but accurate method of evaluation can be derived from eq. (3a) and (3b). After writing $h = q^{(n_2+1)/2} e^{\rho \Delta t/2}$ and adding both equations, one obtains

$$v_1 + v_2 = T_S(h/q + 1/h)/\Delta t$$

Now, $h/q + 1/h$ is less than $h + 1/h$ which is slightly greater than 2 for h near 1. More precisely, we may suppose $h \leq \sqrt{2}$ and then $h + 1/h < 2.122$. So we obtain the approximate formula

$$T_S = \frac{1}{2}(v_1 + v_2) \Delta t \tag{6.6}$$

Once T_S has been calculated, it is easy to solve eq. (4) for ρ. The great advantage of eq. (6) is that ρ is eliminated.

7. Double labelling and FLM

There is a valuable modification of the FLM method in which double labelling with H^3- and C^{14}-thymidine is applied. Counting of labelled mitoses at different times after double labelling provides several FLM curves corresponding to cohorts of differently labelled cells. If the time between C^{14} and H^3 is small (e.g. 1 hour), then the peaks of purely H^3- and purely C^{14}-labelled mitoses are sharp and well separated by troughs at the zero level (Fig.12).

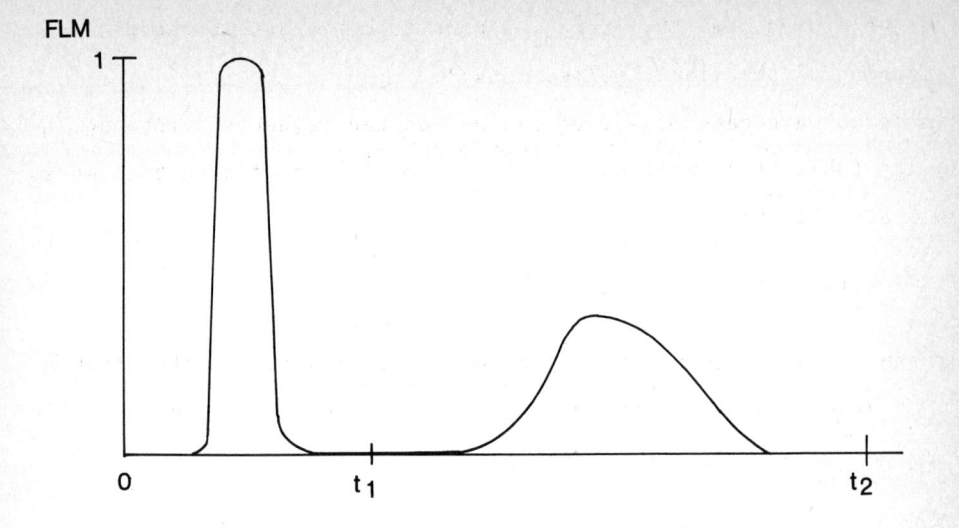

FLM

1

0   t_1 t_2

Fig.12: Fraction of purely C^{14}-labelled mitoses as a function of
time after double labelling.

From these curves one can calculate the mean and the variance of phase durations and cycle time by simple numerical integration. For example, the mean of $T_{G_2} + \frac{1}{2}T_M$ is given by $A^{-1} \int_0^{t_1} t\ FLM(t)dt$, and the mean of the cycle time by $A^{-1} \int_{t_1}^{t_2} t\ FLM(t)dt$ minus the mean of $T_{G_1} + \frac{1}{2}T_M$. Here, A is the area under the corresponding peak. Variances are calculated in a similar way. This method of analysis is independent of any distribution assumption, and therefore it can be used to test hypotheses about the distribution of phase durations. It has been proposed by Schultze, Kellerer and Maurer (1979) in a study of the phase durations of jejunal crypt cells of the mouse. They have shown that in these cells the ratio of mean and standard deviation of T_φ is independent of the phase and that transit times through successive phases are uncorrelated. The assumptions stated in Sec.1. agree with this result.

8. Which experiments are to be chosen?

To conclude this chapter let us review all cell kinetic parameters and the experiments suited to give information about them. For some parameters (e.g. cell loss factor Φ) a combination of experiments is requested.

1) Rate of exponential growth ρ (doubling time $T_d = \log 2 / \rho$)

   Repeated measurements of population size

   Metaphase arrest

   Continuous labelling (with caution)

   Double labelling

2) Cycle time T_C

   Fractions of labelled mitoses

   Double labelling and FLM

   Metaphase arrest (with caution)

   Continuous labelling with metaphase arrest

3) Mitotic time T_M

   Metaphase arrest

4) G_2 phase length T_{G_2}

   Continuous labelling with metaphase arrest

   Fractions of labelled mitoses

5) S phase length T_S

   Continuous labelling

   Fractions of labelled mitoses

   Double labelling

6) G_1 phase length T_{G_1}

    Continuous labelling with metaphase arrest

    Fractions of labelled mitoses

7) Variance of T_C and phases

    Double labelling with C^{14} and H^3 and fractions of labelled mitoses

8) Proliferative fraction (growth fraction) PF

    Continuous labelling with metaphase arrest

    Common method: Determine the index of pulse labelling LI_0, obtain T_S/T_C from the final level of the FLM-curve and apply (1.1b).

9) Loss rate of sterile cells λ

    Continuous labelling

10) Cell loss factor Φ

    Two (hypothetical) cases are to be considered.

  Case a: Only sterile cells are lost

    In this case the equations

    a) $(1-\Phi)$ PF $= \alpha-1$ (3.10, Chap.I)

    b) $I_S = \dfrac{PF}{\alpha-1} e^{\rho T_3}(e^{\rho T_S}-1)$ (5.10, Chap.I)

    c) $\Phi = (2-\alpha) \dfrac{\lambda}{\rho+\lambda}$

    are useful. Equations a) and c) are valid under very general assumptions (Knolle, 1983b). Since I_S is the index of pulse labelling LI_0, we get from a) and b)

$$1-\Phi = \frac{1}{LI_o} e^{\rho T_3} (e^{\rho T_S} - 1)$$

and therefrom Φ can be calculated, if LI_o, ρ, T_S and T_3 are known. If ρ, T_C and PF are known, then we can use $\alpha = \exp(\rho T_C)$ and a) alone. A third possibility is to write a) and c) as a system of two linear equations in Φ and α, which can be solved if ρ, PF and λ are known.

Case b: P-cells and Q-cells are lost at equal rates

Steel (1968) has proposed a method based on the "potential doubling time" and an artificial parameter called λ (see e.g. Gunduz, 1981). A system of 2 equations (1 linear, 1 nonlinear) is derived, which must be solved by iteration, but it is not assured that the iteration process does converge. The experimental data needed are T_d, LI, T_S and T_3.

The author has proposed a simpler method, which requires the same data (Knolle, 1984a). There the equation

$$x = \frac{LI}{T_S} e^{-x(\frac{1}{2}T_S + T_3)}$$

is solved by iteration (convergence is assured) and the cell loss factor is then obtained from $\Phi = (x-\rho)/\rho$.

In a recent paper (Knolle 1986), these formulas and eq. (1.1b) have been applied to the calculation of Φ and PF for 65 tumors from data published in Steel's book.

11) Parameters of the extended model of tumor growth.

   These are the 4 parameters a_{11}, a_{12}, a_{21}, a_{22} of the system
   of equations (4.1 a/b) of Chapter I. When PF and T_S are known,
   a_{12} can be determined from a double-labelling experiment described in Sec. 4 of Chapter III. Continuous-labelling data can
   be evaluated according to the equation

$$1 - CL_t = c\ e^{(a_{22}-\rho)t}$$

   which is derived in the same way as eq.(2.3). This leads to
   the determination of a_{22} if ρ is known. Finally, a_{11} and a_{21}
   are calculated from eq.(4.6), where $r = 1/PF - 1$.

III. CELL KINETICS AND CANCER THERAPY

Introduction

It is a well-established fact that the cytotoxicity of radiation and
of most anticancer drugs depends on cell kinetic parameters (Sinclair
1967, Mendelsohn 1975, Valeriote and v. Putten 1975, Bhuyan 1977).
This has suggested the idea of exploiting kinetic differences between
neoplastic and sensitive normal tissues in order to achieve selective
cell kill, i.e. killing a great fraction of tumor cells while sparing
the normal cells of the renewal tissues (bone marrow, epithelium of
the small intestine, skin). Indeed, cell kinetics are a corner-stone
of many theoretical concepts in the treatment of cancer by radiation
or cytotoxic drugs (Frei et al. 1969, Skipper and Perry 1970, Skipper
1971, Clarkson 1974, Klein and Lennartz 1974, Southwest Oncology Group
1974, Withers 1975, Valeriote and Edelstein 1977, Gerecke 1979, Swan
1980, Smets 1983). Some attempts to design therapy schedules on a rational basis with cell kinetic concepts have failed in practice and
consequently the optimism of the period about 1970 has been displaced
by skepticism (v. Putten, 1974) about the benefit of cell kinetics
for therapy. But recently this approach has become favored again.
There has been a careful palpating of the possibilities and limits
of cytokinetic theory in clinical practice (Langen 1980) and the con-
viction that early failures should be attributed to the lack of data
rather than to a presumed inconsistency of cell kinetic theory (Pallavicini et al. 1982).

Exposure to radiation or anticancer drugs can produce a number of different effects on cells:

1) death of exposed cells

2) death of descendants of exposed cells

3) sterilization of exposed cells

4) retardation or block of the cell cycle

5) recruitment of resting cells to proliferation.

It is accepted that recruitment is not a direct effect but a response of an inherent regulation mechanism to extensive cell loss. The blocking effect is often related to the cell kill effect: if cells are blocked for a long time then they die, and an agent which at low doses causes only block, may cause cell death at high doses. A retardation or block of the cell cycle is caused by some type of sublethal damage, which may be repaired if exposure is stopped in time. Repair of sublethal damage after irradiation has been demonstrated by Elkind (1967).

An agent which causes one or more of the effects 1) - 4) will be called cytotoxic. A secondary effect of many cytotoxic agents is synchronization or at least a perturbation of the stable age distribution: retardation of the cell cycle in a certain phase causes accumulation of cells in this phase, recruitment of resting cells causes a sudden increase in the number of cells in phase G_1 and an agent which kills only cells in a certain phase (phase-specific cell kill) makes the smooth curve of the stable age distribution fall abruptly to zero in the sensitive phase. Synchronization and other kinetic effects may be exploited for cancer therapy by careful timing of drug applications and radiation doses.

It is our goal in this chapter to achieve a quantitative description of cytotoxic and of recruitment effects which may help to improve the treatment of cancer by radiation or drugs. For this sake it is necessary

a) to build mathematical models of the action of cytotoxic agents

b) to review experimental methods which are suited to determine the parameters of the models

c) to develop guide lines for the rational design of therapy schedules based on cell kinetic data.

The first step on this way will be to establish dose-effect relations for single doses, and this requires an exact definition of the effect in quantitative terms. Usually the effects 1) - 3) are measured jointly with a colony test. This is an experiment directed to determine the number n_1 of treated cells and the number n_0 of cells of an untreated control group, which after isolation and incubation in a new medium produce a growing colony of descendants. The ratio n_1/n_0 is called the surviving fraction (SF). In this definition it is assumed (if effect 2) is present) that after a due incubation time, growing colonies can be distinguished from abortive colonies which don't continue to grow (Trott, 1972). Note that sterile cells of the control group do not contribute to n_0, while G_0 cells (which are resting but not sterile) may be stimulated to produce a colony by the procedure of isolation and incubation.

The effect of cytotoxic agents on normal bone marrow stem cells and on leukemic cells in vivo can be studied with the spleen-colony assay. This method exploits the fact that these cells are able to form colonies in the spleen of lethally irradiated mice. More details on colony tests are found in the book by Steel (1977).

In a study on the effect of ara-C in vivo, Fietkau et al. (1984) have employed a method, where the amount of cell kill is determined from the observation of necrotic cells. This method is especially adapted to the study of phase-specific cell kill and will be considered in Section 2. The measurement of retardation and recruitment will be treated in Section 3 and 4. Thereafter, a mathematical model which integrates phase-specific cell kill, retardation of the cell cycle, recruitment of resting cells and pharmacokinetics into the cell kinetic model of Takahashi will be described (Section 5). Computer simulations and recommendations for drug testing and cancer therapy derived from cell kinetics will be presented in Section 6 and 7.

1. The surviving fraction after a single dose

The effect of radiation on cells has been described with much detail,
qualitatively and quantitatively, and several mathematical models,
e.g. the multi-hit and the multi-target model have been developed
(Kellerer and Hug 1972, Swan 1981). The dose of radiation is the reference point in all these models, and theoretical as well as empirical dose-effect relations have been established. If the action of drugs
in vivo is considered, the situation becomes more complex, because
the transport of the drug to the site of the target cells must be considered, which implies that there is only an indirect relation between
dose and effect. The natural approach to this problem is to begin with
the concentration-effect relation, to continue with pharmacokinetic
considerations, and to treat the dose-effect relation at the end.

In a formal manner we may consider cells as molecules of another com-
pound which reacts with the drug and is able to bind an arbitrary number of drug molecules. Let $C(t)$ be the concentration of the drug at
the time t and let Z_i be the number of cells which have bound exactly i drug molecules ($i = 0,1,2,\ldots$). The law of mass action which gov-
erns chemical reactions says that the velocity of the reaction $A + B \rightarrow C$
is proportional to the product of the concentrations of A and B. The
binding of drug molecules by cells may be considered as a sequence
of simultaneous reactions, where the i-th reaction step consists in
adding a new molecule of drug to a cell which has bound already i-1
molecules. The velocity of the 1st step is, according to the law of
mass action, $kC(t)Z_0(t)$ and therefore

$$dZ_0/dt = -k\,C(t)Z_0 \tag{1.1a}$$

where k is the reaction rate constant. Let us suppose that the probability of binding one more molecule does not depend on the number of
molecules already bound, i.e. that all reaction steps have equal velocity. Then the velocity of the i-th reaction is $k\,C(t)\,Z_{i-1}(t)$ and
hence

$$dZ_i/dt = k\,C(t)\,(Z_{i-1}-Z_i) \qquad i=1,2,\ldots \qquad (1.1b)$$

In these equations cell proliferation has been neglected. Let us suppose that a cell dies or produces an abortive colony if and only if
it has bound more than n molecules of drug. Then the SF can be calculated in the following way. If drug action begins at $t=0$ and N_0 cells
are present at $t=0$, then we solve the system of differential equations
(1a/b) with the initial conditions $Z_0(0)=N_0$, $Z_i(0)=0$ ($i=1,2,\ldots$). The
surviving cells are those which never bind more than n molecules, and
hence the SF is given by

$$SF = \frac{1}{N_0} \lim_{t\to\infty} \sum_{i=0}^{n} Z_i(t) \qquad (1.2)$$

Since the differential equations are linear, the solution depends
linearly on the initial conditions and SF is independent on N_0, the
number of cells exposed to the drug. This is the famous fractional-
kill hypothesis introduced by Skipper which says that a certain dose
of a cytotoxic drug kills a certain fraction of the cells exposed
(Skipper, 1964).

With the initial conditions indicated the system (1a/b) has the solution

$$Z_0(t) = N_0 \exp(-k \int_0^t C(s)ds)$$

$$Z_i(t) = \frac{N_0}{i!} (k \int_0^t C(s)ds)^i \exp(-k \int_0^t C(s)ds)$$

and therefore

$$\lim_{t \to \infty} Z_i(t) = \frac{N_o}{i!} \left(k \int_0^\infty C(t)dt \right)^i \exp\left(-k \int_0^\infty C(t)dt\right) \qquad (1.3)$$

This relation exhibits the importance of the area under the concentration curve $AUC = \int_0^\infty C(t)dt$.

In Sec.3 of the Appendix it is shown that AUC is proportional to the dose D. Therefore from eq. (2) and (3) we deduce

$$SF = (1 + fD + \ldots + \frac{1}{n!} f^n D^n)e^{-fD} \qquad (1.4)$$

where f is a constant that depends on the sensitivity of the cells, on the route of administration and pharmacokinetic parameters. This relation is also obtained from the multi-hit model of radiation effect. If only one drug molecule is sufficient to kill a cell (n=0), then

$$SF = e^{-fD} \qquad (1.4a)$$

If fD is small, we may neglect higher terms in (4) and write

$$SF = (1 + fD)e^{-fD}$$
$$\log(1 + fD) = fD - \frac{1}{2}(fD)^2$$
$$\log SF = -\frac{1}{2}(fD)^2$$

Therefore the dose-survival curve in a semilogarithmic plot is close to a parabola, at least in the region of small doses. Fig.1 shows the survival curves for synchronized cells irradiated in different phases of the cell cycle. It is seen that cells in mitosis and G_2 are most sensitive and that some curves are nearly straight lines ($\log SF = -fD$) while others tend to the parabolic type.

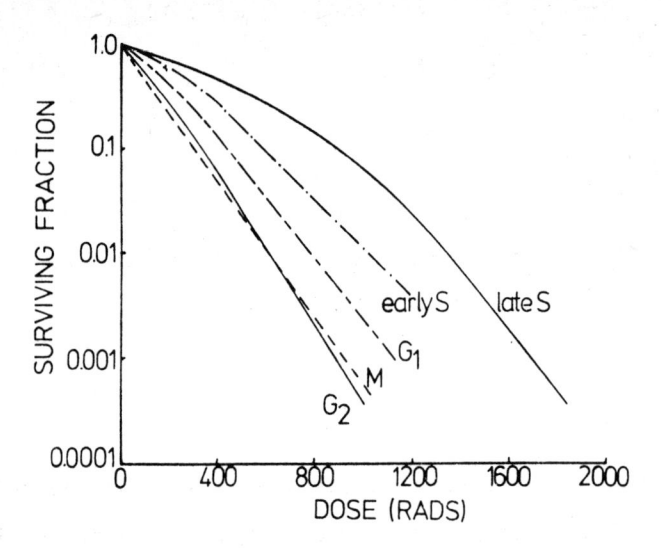

Fig.1: Relation between radiation dose and surviving fraction
      (from Sinclair, 1967).

The formulae derived so far are not valid, if there is a subpopulation
of resistant cells. In this case the effect of prolonged exposure depends on whether the resistant cells can pass to the sensitive subpopulation or not. If r is the fraction of resistant cells and if there
is no passage, then the dose-survival curve approaches the horizontal
line SF = r or log SF = log r as D increases more and more. Furthermore
the dose-survival curve is independent on the time interval, during
which the cells are exposed to effective concentrations of the drug.

Resting cells are resistant to most cytotoxic agents. Furthermore many
agents are phase-specific, i.e. they kill cells with phase-dependent
rates or only in one phase of the cell cycle. An ideal phase-specific
drug kills cells only in one phase of the cell cycle, and even at very
high doses it kills only a fraction of cells equal to the index of
the sensitive phase, if exposure is short. But if the drug doesn't

block the cell cycle, all cycling cells enter the sensitive phase after short or long, and there they are killed if an effective concentration of drug is maintained long enough (Fig.2). The situation is similar, if the drug kills only cycling cells and if recruitment of resting cells into the cycle occurs.

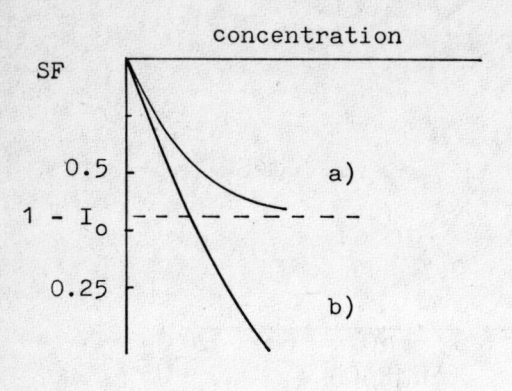

Fig.2: Concentration-survival curve for agent killing cells in
one phase with index I_o
a) short exposure
b) long exposure

In the deduction of eq. (4) we have already seen the importance of the area under the concentration curve (AUC). Now we define the "mean residence time" of the drug:

$$MRT = \frac{1}{AUC} \int_0^\infty tC(t)\,dt$$

MRT corresponds to the exposure time in experiments in vitro. For the frequently-used concentration curves

$$C(t) = c\,e^{-at} \quad \text{(simple elimination) and}$$

$$C(t) = c\,\frac{b}{b-a}\,(e^{-at} - e^{-bt}) \quad \text{(Bateman function)}$$

a simple calculation shows that

$$MRT = \frac{1}{a} \qquad \text{resp.} \qquad MRT = \frac{1}{a} + \frac{1}{b}.$$

The preceding considerations suggest that the surviving fraction for phase-specific drugs decreases with MRT. This presumption has been confirmed by a series of computer simulations with the program CELLU (see Sec.5). The cases of intravenous and of oral application have been considered and modelled by the functions just mentioned. The results are shown in Table 1. It is seen that for AUC=9 the increase of MRT from 1 to 3 and from 3 to 7 h causes a division of the SF by a factor greater than 5.

route	a	b	MRT	AUC			
				1.5	3	6	9
i.v.	1	-	1 h	0.39	0.24	0.152	0.120
oral	1	1/2	3 h	0.34	0.15	0.047	0.022
oral	1	1/6	7 h	0.33	0.11	0.018	0.004
i.v.	1/6	-	6 h	0.37	0.15	0.030	0.009
oral	1/6	1/2	8 h	0.32	0.11	0.016	0.003
oral	1/6	1/6	12 h	0.33	0.11	0.014	0.002

Table 1: Surviving fraction of cells of the leukemia L1210 after a single dose of an S-phase specific agent for different values of AUC and MRT, calculated with the computer program CELLU. In colums 2 and 3 the rates of elimination and invasion are given. The cell kinetic parameters are $T_{G1}=1.6$, $T_S=8.2$, $T_{G2}=1.9$, $T_M=0.5$.

2. Phase specific cell kill

Phase specific cell kill can be detected in vitro, if a synchronous cell population is exposed to the agent at various times, which correspond to various positions of the synchronous wave of cells in the cycle, and the surviving fraction is determined for each time of exposure. Older techniques of cell synchronization are reviewed by Nias and Fox (1971).

The evaluation of this experiment requires the knowledge of the phase durations and is easy if the decay of synchrony is slow. If synchrony is lost rapidly, then the experiment should be modified in the following way: Suppose that a synchronous cell population or cohort has been obtained by mitotic selection at time t=0. Then the cytocidal effect of any agent on cells in G_1 can be assessed in the usual way after exposure of the cohort, say at t=1 hr. The fraction of cells killed, if the cohort is exposed at $t=T_{G_1}+\frac{1}{2}T_S$, should express the kill of cells in S, but there may be a considerable number of cells in G_1 and G_2 due to the variation of T_{G_1} and T_S, and this would lead to an underestimation of S-phase toxicity, if G_1 or G_2 were resistant. Therefore it is better to expose at $t=T_{G_1}+\frac{1}{4}T_S$ and to add a second agent which is already known to be G_1-phase specific and which is neither synergistic or antagonistic with respect to the first. At the time of exposure only few cells will be in G_2, and the cells in G_1 are killed by the second agent, such that the decay of synchrony is partially reversed. In a similar way the effect on cells in G_2 can be assessed.

In any case a high initial degree of synchrony is necessary in order to assess differential sensitivity of the phases. Since this cannot be achieved in vivo (see Sec.7), the demonstration of phase specific cell kill in vivo needs another method, e.g. a labelling technique.

Fietkau, Friede and Maurer-Schultze (1984) demonstrated the phase-specific action of cytosine arabinoside (ara-C) in vivo with the following experiment. Mice bearing the L1210 ascites tumor ($T_{G_1}=4$ hr, $T_S=10$ hr, $T_{G_2M}=1$ hr, PF=1) received H^3-Thymidine at t=-2.5 hr, C^{14}-Thymidine at t=-0.5 hr, and ara-C at t=0hr. This leads to a 2-hr-wide subpopulation of purely C^{14}-labelled cells in early S-phase and a 2-hr-wide subpopulation of purely H^3-labelled cells in G_2-, M- and early G_1-phase. The remaining cells in S are double labelled (8-hr-wide), and the remaining cells in G_1 are unlabelled (3-hr-wide). The fate of the differently labelled populations can be followed up by means of double-layer autoradiographs. The percentage of purely C^{14}- and double labelled cells decreases, that of purely H^3-labelled cells increases, and the percentage of unlabelled cells oscillates (Fig.3).

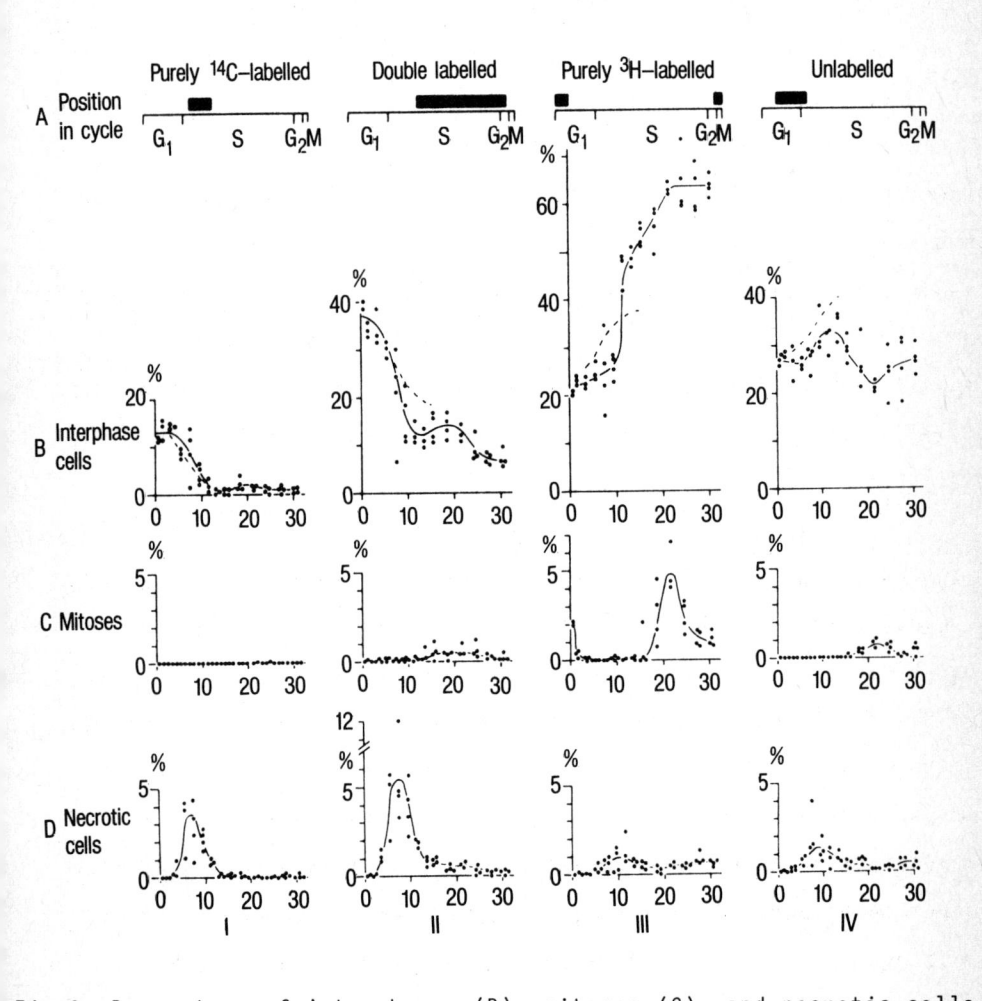

Fig.3: Percentage of interphases (B), mitoses (C), and necrotic cells (D) for the differently labelled subpopulations as a function of time after ara-C application (from Fietkau et al., 1984).

From this result it can be inferred intuitively that the S-phase is more sensitive than the other phases. More precise information is obtained through the count of necrotic cells and mathematical evaluation of the data on the basis of a compartment model.

Cells that are destined to die pass through a transient state, which has typical morphological features and is called necrosis. Fietkau et al. represent the flow of cells through necrosis to disappearance (Fig.4) by the differential equations

$$dx_1/dt = -d(t) x_1 \qquad\qquad (2.1a)$$

$$dx_2/dt = d(t) x_1 - \gamma x_2 \qquad\qquad (2.1b)$$

where x_1 (x_2) is the number of vital (necrotic) cells. The constant γ is the rate of disappearence of necrotic cells and $d(t)$ is the probability per unit of time of a vital cell to become necrotic.

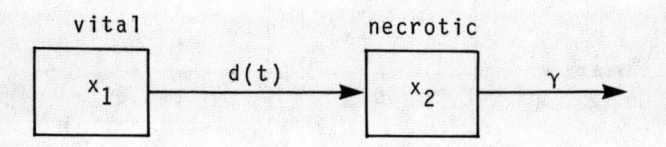

Fig.4: Flow of cells through necrosis to disappearance

The design of the experiment (count of vital and necrotic cells in samples taken at different times) implies, that only the ratio x_2/x_1 can be observed directly. But the absolute numbers x_1, x_2 and the function $d(t)$ can be estimated from the data in the following way. From (1 a/b) one deduces

$$d = \frac{(r' + \gamma)r}{1 + r}$$

where $r = x_2/x_1$ and $r' = dr/dt$. A guessed value of γ is inserted, r and

r' are obtained from the observations, and then the differential equations (1 a/b) are solved and the calculated values of x_2/x_1 are compared with the observed values. This procedure is repeated with various values of γ until the best fit to the data is obtained.

The model (1 a/b) can be applied immediately to the subpopulations
where no cell division is occuring during the observation period. Since
the mitotic index falls from about 2% to less than 0.3% during the
1st hour and stays there for about 10 hours, cell division may be neglected entirely. If this is accepted, the function d(t) can be determined separately for each of the differently labelled subpopulations.
For the sake of simplicity Fietkau et al. have aggregated purely C^{14}-
labelled with double labelled and purely H^3-labelled with unlabelled
cells. The first group are the cells initially in S and G_2, the second
group contains the rest. The calculated values of d(t) are given in
Table 2.

Time after ara-C	Probability of becoming necrotic in phase	
	M and G_1	S and G_2
0	0.00	0.00
2	0.01	0.01
4	0.02	0.12
6	0.03	0.215
8	0.04	0.244
10	0.01	0.23
12	0.01	0.09
14	0.01	0.06

Table 2: The function d(t) from eqs. (1 a/b) for different phases
of the cell cycle (Fietkau, unpublished data)

Eq. (1a) is similar to eq. (1.1a), but the functions d(t) and C(t) are
quite distinct. Since the first necrotic cells appear hours after the
rise of the concentration curve, we have d(t)=0 during several hours

of drug exposure. In the model of this section the SF is the fraction
of cells that stay in x_1 for ever, i.e. SF $= \lim_{t \to \infty} x_1(t)/x_1(0)$ or

$$SF = \exp\left(-\int_0^\infty d(t)dt\right)$$

If we calculate the integral with the trapezoidal rule, truncating
at t=14 and using the values of Table 2, we obtain SF $= 0.78$ for M/G_1
and SF $= 0.16$ for S/G_2.

These data will be used in Section 5 in a simulation study of the
action of ara-C.

3. Block of the cell cycle

The arrest of dividing cells in metaphase by colchicine is an example
of a cytotoxic drug action which blocks the cell cycle at a single
event of short duration. If the concentration of the blocking agent
is high enough, then each cell which begins metaphase is arrested
there. Furthermore no cell is arrested at another point of the cycle.
Consequently, after due exposure time all proliferating cells are mitotic, and the age distribution shows a sharp peak in mitosis and a
zero level in the phases G_1, S and G_2.

It is necessary to distinguish well between arrest at a point (e.g.
metaphase arrest) and retardation of transit through a phase or sub-
phase. An example of retardation is given by any agent that inhibits
the synthesis of DNA. At a certain concentration the agent inactivates
a certain fraction p of the enzyme which is essential for DNA-synthesis. Since the amount of DNA to be produced is fixed, the duration of
S-phase is inversely proportional to the rate of DNA-synthesis, i.e.

under drug action the S-phase is lengthened by the factor $z=p^{-1}$. This factor is called the retardation factor. It is important to know whether cells recover from the effect of the retarding (blocking) agent immediately after end of exposure or with delay. This question can be answered through the study of the mechanism of action, but also by well-designed kinetic experiments. The time between end of exposure and release of retarded cells to normal proliferation is called the recovery time. It is also important to distinguish between cells that retain full reproductive ("clonogenic") capacity during retardation, and those retarded cells that have lost the capacity of producing a colony of descendants (Camplejohn, 1980). One has to be aware of this, if retardation in S is to be measured by an increase of the S-phase index. If many retarded cells are in fact destined to die, then the fraction of clonogenic cells in S is not equal to the index of pulse labelling and must be determined by different methods (Gray, 1983).

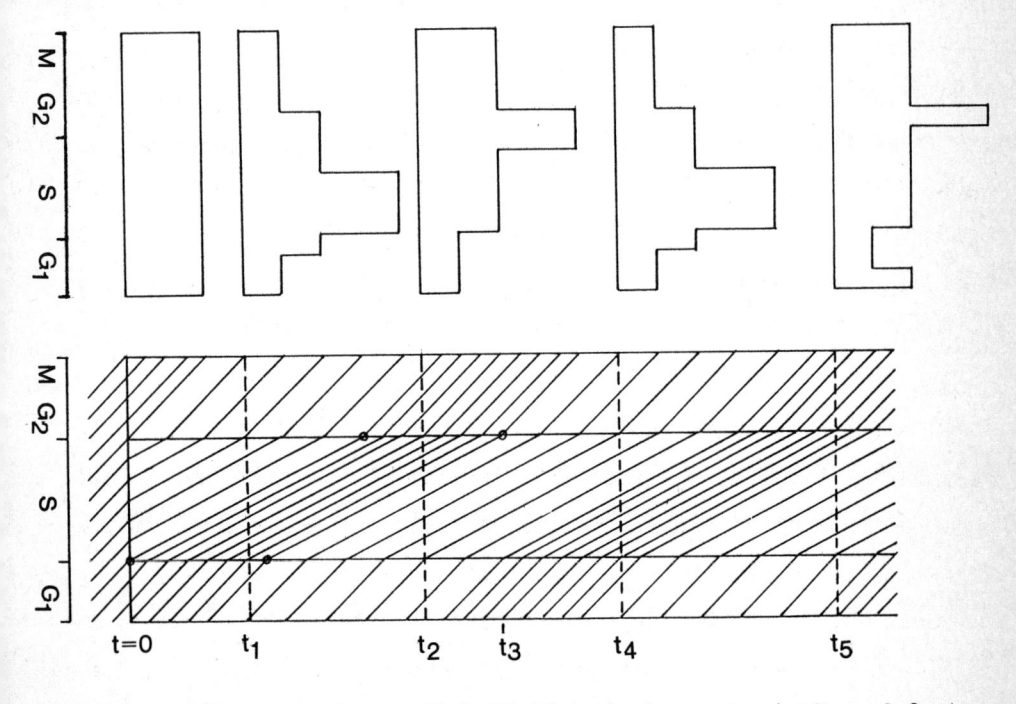

Fig.5: Oscillations of age distribution during retardation of S-phase

The retardation factor can be incorporated into the model with uniform cycle time (phase durations) and into the Takahashi model as well. In the latter model retardation (block) is expressed by decrease (vanishing) of the passage rate.

The response of a cell population to a retarding agent is a rather complex phenomenon. This will already become evident if we consider only a steady state population with uniform cycle time T_C. Suppose that cells in vitro are exposed to a constant concentration of an agent which retards the S-phase by the factor 2. We represent the life cycle of a cell by a line in the plane with coordinates time and maturity (functional age): a cell with age a at time t occupies the point with coordinates a and t. The untreated cells have a straight life line with slope 1. From the beginning of treatment (t=0) that part of the life line that belongs to the S-phase, has slope 1/2 (Fig.5). The age density at time t_i is represented by the density of life lines intersecting the line $t=t_i$ (Fig.5, upper part). At the left of the line t=0 all life lines have slope 1 and the density of lines is equal in G_1, S, G_2 and M. Beginning at t=0, the slope of the lines through S is 1/2, cells are accumulated in S and the density is reduced in G_2 and M and ultimately in G_1 (t=t_1). But the cells accumulated in S must pass to G_2, and therefore the age density in G_2 rises again (t=t_2). Between t_1 and t_3 the flow of cells into S is reduced and so the S-phase index falls again to the initial level (t=t_3). At t=t_4 the same state as at t=t_1 is attained again. Thus the response to constant concentration of the agent is an infinite succession of undamped oscillations. The period of the oscillations is T_C+T_S, since the length of S-phase is doubled.

In the past many people have believed that the decrease after the first peak of the fraction of cells in the retarded phase must be attributed to deficiency in the performance of the drug. This view is clearly rejected by the preceding analysis.

When there is a distribution of cycle times, then the situation is similar, with the difference that a new stable age distribution is approached through damped oscillations. This is a direct consequence of the general law of decay of sychrony (Sec.6, Chap.I). It should be remarked at this point, that a cell population with constant kinetic parameters has a unique stable age distribution which depends only on these parameters. If the kinetic parameters are changed (e.g. by delay of the progression of cells through a phase), then the stable age distribution is changed too. Moreover, a population which is asynchronous with respect to one stable age distribution, is partially synchronous with respect to the other. This implies that any abrupt change of parameters provokes a track of damped oscillations. In particular, when exposure to a retarding agent is stopped, a second track of oscillations is induced which superposes the first track originating from start of exposure (Fig.6).

In vivo, the situation is even more complicated, because the concentration of the drug is changing at any moment. A comprehensive mathematical model and computer calculations are necessary in order to simulate the response of cell populations to retarding agents in vivo. Nevertheless, the maximum of the index $\tilde{I}_\varphi$ of the retarded phase can be calculated approximately by the simple method depicted in Fig.5. Due to decay of synchrony the true maximum will be a little bit smaller than the value which will be deduced under the assumption of uniform cycle time T_C. Suppose that the phase with duration T_φ is retarded by the factor z, and denote the duration of the phases preceding and following it with T_1 and T_3. The densely shaded parallelogram in Fig.5, whose vertices are marked by circles, has the basis $T_1 + T_3 = T_C - T_\varphi$ and its upper left vertex is on the line $t = zT_\varphi$. Intersection with a vertical line between $t = T_C - T_\varphi$ and $t = zT_\varphi$

results in a cross section equal to $(T_C-T_\varphi)/z$.

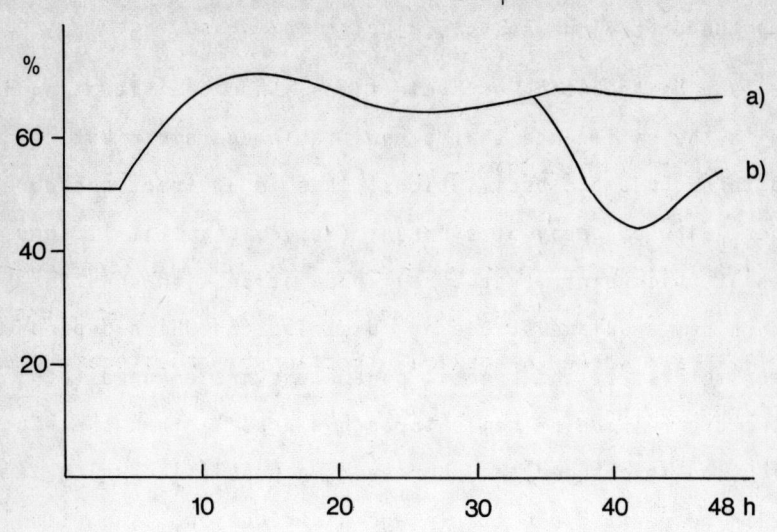

Fig.6: Oscillations of S-phase index after change of kinetic parameters, calculated with the computer program CELLU.
a) T_S is doubled at t=4h. b) T_S is doubled at t=4h and set
to normal value at t=34h. Constancy of index indicates a
stable, asynchronous age distribution. T_C = 15h, T_S = 8h.

Referring to cell density the section of length $(T_C-T_\varphi)/z$ which belongs to the densely shaded area, is to be weighted with the factor
z, while the rest of the phase, with length $T_\varphi-(T_C-T_\varphi)/z$, has weight
1. Therefore, if $T_C-T_\varphi \leqq z\,T_\varphi$, the maximal number of cells in the retarded phase is proportional to

$$(T_C-T_\varphi) + T_\varphi - \frac{1}{z}(T_C-T_\varphi) = (1-\frac{1}{z})T_C + \frac{1}{z}T_\varphi$$

This is to be divided through T_C and multiplied by PF, in order to
obtain the maximum of the phase index $\tilde{I}_\varphi$ during retardation:

$$\max \tilde{I}_\varphi = (1-\frac{1}{z})PF + \frac{1}{z}\frac{T_\varphi}{T_C} PF$$

Now, in an untreated, non-growing population the age distribution is rectangular and $(T_\varphi/T_C)PF$ is the value of the phase index I_φ, and we obtain

$$\max \tilde{I}_\varphi = (1-\frac{1}{z})PF + \frac{1}{z}I_\varphi \tag{3.1}$$

The condition $T_C-T_\varphi \leq z\,T_\varphi$ is usually satisfied for the long phases S and G_1. If $z\,T_\varphi < T_C-T_\varphi$, then the maximal densely shaded cross section is all T_φ and hence the maximal fraction of proliferating cells in the retarded phase is $z\,T_\varphi/T_C$ and

$$\max \tilde{I}_\varphi = z\,I_\varphi \tag{3.2}$$

Both formulae have been deduced for non-growing populations, but also in the case of growth they are in fair agreement with results of calculations with the computer program CELLU. These formulae can be used to calculate z, if $\max(\tilde{I}_\varphi)$ is known as well as T_φ and T_C. It is sufficient to represent the relation between z and $\max(\tilde{I}_\varphi)$ geometrically for $z \geq 1$. If $2T_\varphi \geq T_C$ then only eq. (1) applies. In the opposite case eq. (2) applies for $1 \leq z \leq T_C/T_\varphi-1$, and eq. (1) else (Fig.7).

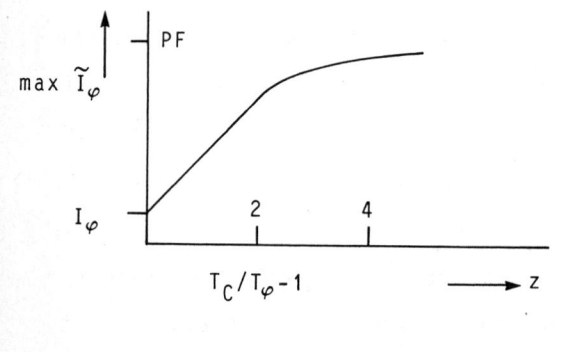

Fig.7: Maximum of phase index as a function of retardation factor z for $T_C/T_\varphi = 3$

In the introduction to this chapter it has been mentioned that many agents cause block or retardation and cell kill as well. When this is the case, it is an important question whether retardation occurs immediately before, during, or after the phase, where cells are killed. In the first case a fraction of those cells, which at the beginning of exposure are in the resistant phases, does not enter the sensitive phase during the exposure period. These cells are protected by the action of the cytocidal agent itself - a phenomenon called "self-limited cell kill." In the second case cell kill increases with duration of exposure.

Ara-C and hydroxyurea are drugs that kill cells selectively in S and arrest cells temporarily in G_1. v. Putten (1974) writes that "if the killing of normal tissue cells by these drugs is self-limited, prolonged exposure should not be unduly toxic." But "for ara-C the occurrence of bone marrow damage seems ... more related to the duration of exposure than to the dose." Therefore, he concludes that this is an example where "cell kinetic principles and observations on the intact organism point in ... clearly opposite directions." However, a paper by Bhuyan et al. (1973) suggests that there is indeed no contradiction between cell kinetics and clinical medicine, so far as self-limited cell kill by ara-C and hydroxyurea is concerned. The authors report an experiment with DON-cells (fibroblasts of the Chinese hamster) synchronized by mitotic selection, plated and then exposed to ara-C (hydroxyurea) for 1 h beginning at 0, 1, 2, 3h after plating. The SF was determined in each case and compared with the SF obtained when the drug was added immediately after plating (i.e. in mitosis or early G_1) and left in contact during the period of experiment (Fig. 8). About 75% of the cells exposed from 0 to 4h and about 25% of the cells exposed from 3 to 4h survived. From the difference of 45% they concluded that the progression through G_1 of cells exposed from 0 to 4h had been retarded by the drug. On the other hand there is no complete block of the G_1/S transition, since 30% of these cells have been killed. Now, if the concept of complete block is replaced by that of retardation, then the observation of increased bone marrow damage agrees well with these observations in vitro and cell kinetic principles.

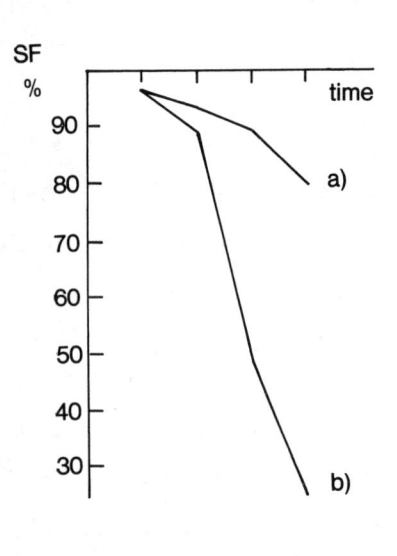

Fig.8: Effect of retardation in G_1 on survival of cells exposed to ara-C. a: drug was added to mitotic cells immediately after plating and was left in contact. Cell survival was determined at 1,2,3,4h after plating. b: mitotic cells were plated and exposed to drug for 1h at 0,1,2,3h after plating. After drug exposure cell survival was determined. (From Bhuyan et al., 1973)

Through the foregoing considerations it has become evident that the assessment of simultaneous retardation and cell kill is a difficult task. Therefore we treat at first the retardation effect alone. If only one phase is affected and the index of this phase is observed for some time during drug exposure at constant concentration, then the retardation factor z can be calculated from eq. (1) or eq. (2). With respect to the phases G_1 and G_2 there is the problem that they cannot be distinguished neither by morphology nor by autoradiography. This limitation has been overcome by flow microfluorometry. The determination of the DNA content of single cells by this method and the analysis of the distribution of DNA content provides values of the fraction of cells in G_1, in G_2 and M, and in different stages of S-phase. The method has become an important tool in the study of retardation, but it can be applied only to single-cell suspensions. Therefore we will describe two methods, one for G_1 and one for G_2, which use only counts of mitoses and labelling indices.

A. Retardation in G_1

An asynchronous cell population is simultaneously and continuously exposed to colchicine (or some other blocker of mitosis), H^3-Thymidine and the agent to be tested (Wheeler et al., 1972). The labelling index is determined at various times during exposure. A control population is exposed only to colchicine and H^3-Thymidine. If the labelling index of the test population grows slower than that of the control, retardation in G_1 is evident. The use of a blocker of mitosis is intended to prevent that the number of labelled cells is increased by cell division rather than by passage of unlabelled cells from G_1 to S.

The labelling index of the control population is given in eq. (4.1) of Chap.II. Since in the population exposed to the drug the progression of cells through G_1 is retarded by the factor z, the broken line in Fig.8 (Chap.II) which limits the area of labelled cells is at the distance t/z from the G_1/S border, i.e. t is to be replaced by t/z and

$$CL_t = e^{\rho T_3}\{e^{\rho(t/z+T_S)} - 1\}$$

Using the approximation (5.9) of Chap.I and neglecting the factor $\exp(\frac{1}{2}\rho t)$ resp. $\exp(\frac{1}{2}\rho t/z)$ we obtain

$$CL_t \simeq \rho(t + T_S)E \qquad \text{(control)} \qquad (3.3)$$

$$CL_t \simeq \rho(\frac{t}{z} + T_S)E \qquad \text{(drug)} \qquad (3.4)$$

where $E = \exp\{\rho(T_3 + \frac{1}{2}T_S)\}$. Therefore a plot of both indices of continuous labelling over time results in straight lines with slope ρE resp. $\rho E/z$. This is a way to determine the retardation factor z.

B. Retardation in G_2

An analogous experiment, without labelling and with observation of mitotic instead of labelling index, is proposed for G_2. We have seen in the section on metaphase arrest, that the increase of I_M is resp. given by

$$I_M(t) = \frac{PF}{T_C}(t + T_M - t_1) \qquad\qquad (\rho = 0)$$

$$\log(1 + I_M(t)) = \rho(t + T_M - t_1) \qquad\qquad (\rho > 0)$$

where t_1 is the time from metaphase to end of mitosis. Again we have to replace t by t/z on the right side, accounting for retardation now in G_2. Comparing the slope of the plotted I_M resp. $\log(1 + I_M)$ observed sequentially in the treated and the control population, the retardation factor z is readily obtained. If T_{G_2} and z are small, cells initially in S may soon reach mitosis. Therefore the period of observation must not exceed 2h, if $T_{G_2} \leqq 1h$ and if z is expected to be $\leqq 2$.

The difficulty inherent in the investigation of simultaneous retardation and cell kill has already been announced. As an example we consider the problem of how retardation in S can be demonstrated in the presence of S-phase specific cell kill. Karon and Shirakawa (1970) proposed an experiment with continuous and pulse labelling and argued, that "the rate of passage from S to G_2" is equal to the difference between the index of continuous and that of pulse labelling. Since this difference is greater in the control than in the treated population, they conclude that ara-C interferes with the passage of cells from S to G_2.

In order to check whether this is correct, let us use the following denotations:

S_t number of cells in S at time t

N_t number of all cells at time t

S_{in} number of cells that entered S during $(t-\Delta t, t)$

S_{out} number of cells that left S during $(t-\Delta t, t)$

S_d number of S-cells that died during $(t-\Delta t, t)$

Then we can write

$$LI_t = \frac{S_{t-\Delta t} + S_{in} - S_{out} - S_d}{N_t} \tag{3.5}$$

$$CL_t = \frac{S_{t-\Delta t} + S_{in} - S_d}{N_t} \tag{3.6}$$

In the Takahashi model the passage rate a_i refers to the compartment K_i and is defined correctly as the fraction

$$\frac{\text{number of cells leaving } K_i}{\Delta t \cdot \text{number of cells in } K_i}$$

So long as cells are nearly uniformly distributed throughout S-phase, we may define the passage rate from S to G_2 analogously by

$$a_S = \frac{S_{out}}{S_t} \Delta t^{-1}$$

Now we deduce from (5) and (6)

$$CL_t - LI_t = \frac{S_{out}}{N_t} = \frac{S_{out}}{S_t} \cdot \frac{S_t}{N_t} = a_S \cdot LI_t \cdot \Delta t$$

and hence the passage rate at time t is

$$a_S = \frac{CL_t - LI_t}{LI_t} \, \Delta t^{-1} \qquad\qquad (3.7)$$

and not $(CL_t - LI_t) \, \Delta t^{-1}$ as assumed by Karon and Shirakawa (1970).
Therefore the statement of these authors that ara-C should retard the
passage from S to G_2, is doubtful. Nevertheless their experiment, if
adequately evaluated, may indeed give information about retardation
in S.

4. Recruitment of resting cells

Since the proliferative fraction of cells grown in culture is always
1 or little below 1, recruitment of resting cells is a cell kinetic
event which can only be studied in vivo. Nevertheless it has been observed rather early, even in clinical situations. Frei et al. (1969)
compared the effect of ara-C given as a single injection and as continuous infusion over periods from 24 to 96 h on the normal human
bone marrow. The degree of bone marrow toxicity (indicated by leuko-
and thrombocytopenia in the peripheral blood) depended strongly on
the duration of exposure, and the toxicity of a single injection was
practically zero, however high the dose was (Fig.9). This observation
was one of the points which should support the claim of v. Putten
(1974) that cell kinetic theories are sometimes conflicting with clinical experience (see Section 3). And in fact it cannot be explained
by the S-phase specificity of the agent and other effects related to

the cell cycle alone. But it is perfectly explained by the following hypotheses, which today can be considered as facts:

a) ara-C kills only proliferating cells

b) at least 80% of the stem cells of human bone marrow are in the resting state before treatment

c) resting stem cells are stimulated to re-enter the cycle by the action of ara-C.

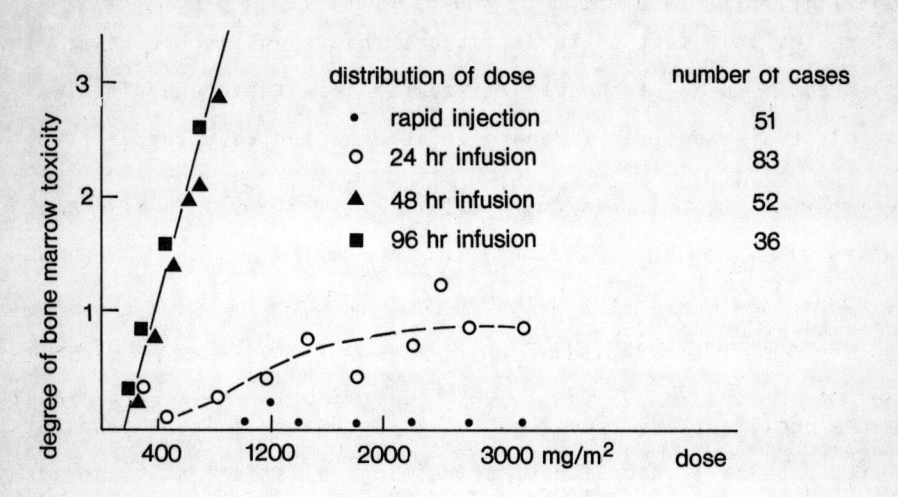

Fig.9: Bone marrow toxicity of cytosine arabinoside in patients (Frei, 1969).

A quantitive study of recruitment in human bone marrow would be an important aid to reduce bone marrow toxicity in cancer chemotherapy without reducing the total dose and has been attempted by Smets et al. (1983). In cell populations in animals, recruitment can be studied by the following double labelling experiment (Korr et al., 1983): Continuous labelling with C^{14}-Thymidine for more than one cycle time leads to C^{14}-labelling of all P-cells. At a time Δt after the end of the continuous C^{14}-TdR application a single dose of H^3-TdR is injected. C^{14}-labelled cells become double-labelled if they are in S at the time of injection, and remain purely C^{14}-labelled else. Resting cells that are recruited and start DNA synthesis after the end of C^{14}-labelling, remain unlabelled until the moment of H^3-labelling and then become purely H^3-labelled, if they are still in S. Thus the number of purely H^3-labelled cells is equal to the number of resting cells recruited during a time interval of length T_S, provided that $\Delta t \geq T_S$ and that recruited unlabelled cells have not yet divided. The latter condition is satisfied if all recruited cells enter the cycle in G_1 and if Δt is smaller than the time spent by the quickest cells in phases S, G_2 and M. Since the duration of S is rather uniform, it is convenient to choose $\Delta t = T_S$.

Now we refer to the extended model of tumor growth proposed in Chap.I. In that model a_{12} is the (constant) rate of recruitment, i.e. $a_{12}Q(t)\Delta t$ is the number of Q-cells recruited in $(t,t+\Delta t)$. If this is divided through the number of all cells and if we use PF=P/(P+Q)=1-Q/(P+Q) then we obtain that $a_{12}(1-PF(t))\Delta t$ is the fraction of Q-cells recruited in $(t,t+\Delta t)$ with respect to all cells. This holds also if a_{12} depends on time. For the sake of simplicity we neglect the time-lag between recruitment and beginning of DNA-synthesis. Therefore, if H^3-labelling is executed at $t=t^*$ then all cells recruited between t^*-T_S and t^* become purely H^3-labelled, and we obtain

$$\text{fraction purely } H^3\text{-labelled} = \int_{t^*-T_S}^{t^*} a_{12}(t)(1-PF(t))dt \qquad (4.1)$$

In the special case when a_{12} and PF are constant, we have

$$\text{fraction purely } H^3\text{-labelled} = a_{12}T_S(1-PF) \qquad (4.1a)$$

This fraction is observed by autoradiography, and therefore a_{12} can be determined if T_S and PF are known.

Recruitment at a constant rate is compatible with exponential growth and constant PF, as has been shown in Chapter I. In contrast, recruitment at an increased rate a_{12} which is caused by some sort of stimulus, implies an elevation of PF with corresponding elevation of the mitotic and the S-phase index. Furthermore, if many resting cells are recruited during a short time, synchronization is observed, because the great majority of recruited cells enters the cycle in one phase, namely in G_1.

Variable rates of recruitment can be measured if the double labelling experiment is repeated several times. Table 3 gives an experimental design for the study of stimulated recruitment in a cell population with $T_C = 15\,h$ and $T_S = 10\,h$, together with hypothetical values of the fraction of purely H^3-labelled cells.

Animal	moment of stimulus	period of C^{14}-label	moment of H^3-label	fraction purely H^3-labelled
1	18 h	0 to 18 h	28 h	$h_1 = 0$
2	13 h	0 to 18 h	28 h	$h_2 = 0.06$
3	8 h	0 to 18 h	28 h	$h_3 = 0.11$
4	3 h	0 to 18 h	28 h	$h_4 = 0.08$

Table 3: Quantitative assay of stimulated recruitment

The fractions h_1, h_2, h_3, h_4 correspond to recruitment during 0 to 10, 5 to 15, 10 to 20, 15 to 25 h after stimulus, respectively. Now let $F_1, F_2, \ldots$ be the interval 0 to 5 h, 5 to 10 h, ... after stimulus and suppose that a_{12} has the constant value f_i during F_i. Then, using eq. (1) and $T_S = 10$ and neglecting the increase of PF, we obtain

$$h_i = 5(f_i + f_{i+1})(1-PF) \qquad i = 1, \ldots, 4$$

Although there are 5 unknowns and only 4 equations, the system can be solved, because $h_1=0$ implies at once $f_1=0$ and $f_2=0$. If e.g. PF=0.8, then $f_3=0.06$, $f_4=0.05$, $f_5=0.03$.

Recruitment can be studied also by H^3-labelling alone. After continuous labelling during a suitable time interval, nearly 100% of the mitoses are labelled permanently, and then resting (unlabelled) cells re-entering the cycle after the outset of labelling will produce a decrease of the fraction of labelled mitoses. This method has been used by Dombernowsky and Bichel (1976).

5. A complex mathematical model and computer programs

In this section we describe a mathematical model of a cell population with proliferating and resting cells which includes the various effects of cytotoxic agents. This model can be used to test hypotheses about the interplay of several cytotoxic effects and to study the influence of each parameter separately. Furthermore, it can account for changes of drug concentration in vivo and can therefore predict the effect of drug elimination rate and route of administration on cell survival.

A flow diagram of the model is presented in Fig.10. The cell cycle is divided into the compartments $K_1,\ldots,K_n$. Mitosis is completed in K_n, and the daughter cells pass to K_1 or to the resting state G_o. Cells in G_o can be recruited into the cycle at a rate which depends on drug concentration. Cells which have been hit by the agent are removed from the cycle and pass through the "hospital" compartment H to necrosis and vanish. The progression through the cell cycle and the passage to H are also controlled by drug concentration.

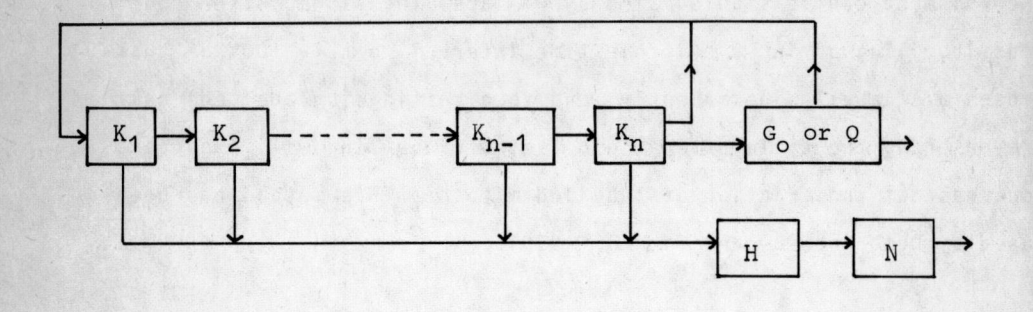

Fig.10: Flow diagram of the mathematical model

The model is constituted by a system of differential equations which are obtained by a suitable modification of the Takahashi equations. Two typical equations of the system have the form

$$dx_i/dt = a_{i-1}x_{i-1} - \frac{a_i}{z_i(t)} x_i - d_i(t)x_i \tag{5.1}$$

$$dx_{i+1}/dt = \frac{a_i}{z_i(t)} x_i - a_{i+1}x_{i+1}$$

Here it has been assumed that only the compartment K_i is affected by cell kill and retardation. The relation between cell kill d_i, retardation z_i and concentration C is given by

$$d_i(t) = D_iC(t) \qquad z_i(t) = 1 + Z_iC(t) \tag{5.2}$$

where D_i and Z_i are constants that express the sensitivity of cells in compartment K_i (i=1,...,n).

Due to the relation for d_i eq. (1) may be interpreted as eq. (1.1a) applied to a single compartment. Indeed, if we consider a situation, where entrance and exit from K_i (cell kill excluded) are balanced, then eq. (1) takes the form

$$dx_i/dt = -d_i(t)x_i = -D_iC(t)x_i$$

and the surviving fraction for cells in K_i is given by

$$SF_i = \exp(-D_i \int_0^\infty C(t)dt) \tag{5.3}$$

The relation for z_i was deduced from a model of inhibition of DNA-synthesis, where the retarding agent reacts with a DNA-related enzyme according to the Michaelis-Menten law.

The compartments H and N are essential, when the model shall describe an experiment in which the drug effect is assessed by the count of vital and necrotic cells. In all other cases they can be omitted. The growth and decay of H and N is described by the differential equations

$$dH/dt = \sum d_i x_i - \beta H$$

$$dN/dt = \beta H - \gamma N$$

where β is a time-dependent function (e.g. the function $d(t)$ from Section 2) and γ is constant. Recruitment of resting cells to compartment K_1 is expressed by addition of the term $Qm_1C/(1+m_2C)$ to the first equation of system (7.5) and by the additional equation

$$dQ/dt = (2-\alpha)a_n x_n - \frac{m_1 C}{1+m_2 C} Q - \lambda_Q Q$$

for the number of resting cells.

The model can describe the combined action of an arbitrary number of
drugs if biochemical synergism as well as antagonism is excluded.
Different effects of the same drug which are not simultaneous (e.g.
cell kill and recruitment), can be treated as unique effects of several fictitious drugs with appropriately delayed concentration curves.

On the basis of this model the computer program CELLU has been con-
structed. It is capable of simulating simultaneous effects of two
drugs, if calculation of the number of necrotic cells is included,
and of three drugs otherwise. The biological and pharmacological data
required as input are:
- mean duration of phases
- number of compartments of each phase (depends on the variance of
  phase duration)
- division factor α
- D_i (i=1,...,n) for each drug (refers to cell kill)
- Z_i (i=1,...,n) for each drug (refers to retardation)
- m_1, m_2 for each drug (refers to recruitment)
- concentration curve of each drug
- function β (transition to necrosis)

The program solves the differential equations of the model with the
improved Euler method. Initial values for the x_i may be chosen arbitrarily or corresponding to the stable age distribution of the unperturbed cell population. The period p, for which the solution is wanted, the number of integration steps ($\leq$ 1000) and the number of lines
of output N_z may be chosen conveniently. Results are printed in a table
containing the total number of cells, the fraction in each phase and,

if wanted, the fraction in selected compartments at N_z equidistant time points between 0 and p.

The structure of the model does not provide the possibility for retardation effects to have a recovery time $t_r > 0$. This can be achieved by a similar model with additional compartments for blocked cells which have to be traversed before return into the cycle. Furthermore, cell kill according to the multi-hit and multi-target model and repair of sublethal damage can be included by several groups of hospital compartments from which return into the cycle is possible. But in view of the lack of empirical data, these more complex models have not been transformed into computer programs.

In its present form the program CELLU is adapted to simulate the effect of one, two or three repeated doses of several drugs. If the number of repetitions becomes greater, as in many therapy schedules, integration with ≤ 1000 steps may confer intolerable numerical errors. Instead of increasing the number of integration steps we have applied the theory of Floquet on linear differential equations with periodic coefficients (see Appendix). The computer program FLOQ is a modification of CELLU for periodically changing drug concentrations on the basis of Floquet's theory. It computes the long term growth rate (decay rate) of a cell population subject to a periodic regimen of drug or radiation applications. The computer program MITO generates the curve of fractions of labelled mitoses if mean and variance of the phase durations are given.

The use of the program CELLU will be illustrated by two examples.

Example 1

The result of the experiment by Bhuyan et al. (see Fig.8) suggested the hypothesis that ara-C and hydroxyurea retard cells in G_1 and kill them in S. The model will support this hypothesis and pronounce it in quantitative terms. The experimental design and the properties of untreated cells determine a part of the input data for the computer simulation, the remaining data have to be guessed. The DON cells used in the experiment have a G_1-phase of 2 h and are in early G_1 at time t=0. More cell kinetic information is not supplied in the paper by Bhuyan et al. (1973). But since the duration of the experiment was 4 h and cells in G_2 and M are not to be expected, T_{G_2}, T_M and the division factor α can be chosen arbitrarily, and to T_S the commonly accepted value 8 h can be assigned. Since the variance of T_{G_1} is not known, four compartments have been assigned arbitrarily to G_1.

Now, the decisive step is to guess the cell kill rate of cells in S. This will be achieved with the aid of the data of Table 4, which contains the percentages of cells in G_1 and in S of the untreated population after 1, 2, 3, 4 h and the percentage K of cells killed by exposure during 1 h beginning at 1, 2, 3 h. The columns G_1 and S have been calculated with the program, the values of column K are taken from Fig.8. If only cells in S are killed, then (S-K)/S is the surviving fraction of cells in S.

time	G_1	S	K	(S-K)/S
0	100	0	-	-
1	86	14	12(?)	0.14
2	43	57	50	0.12
3	15	84	75	0.11
4	5	92	-	-

Table 4: Percentage of cells in phases G_1 and S and of cells killed by ara-C (see text)

It appears that (S-K)/S is rather stable, with a mean of about 0.12. During exposure the concentration of ara-C was $5\mu g/ml$, so that $AUC = \int_0^\infty C(t)dt = 5$. Therefore from eq. (3) we get $SF_i = e^{-5D_i} = 0.12$ or $D_i = 0.4$, if a unique value is assigned to the cell kill rates of all the S-compartments.

The final list of input data contains the following values:

- The phases G_1, S, G_2, M have 4, 4, 1, 1 compartments and their duration is 2, 8, 1, 1 h respectively

- at t=0 all cells are in the 1st compartment

- nonzero cell kill parameters are D_5, ..., D_8=0.4 (S-phase)

- nonzero retardation parameters are Z_1,...,Z_4=0.2 (G_1-phase)

- concentration is 5.0 µg/ml

  1) from t=1 to t=2 h

  2) from t=2 to t=3 h

  3) from t=3 to t=4 h

  4) from t=0 to t=3 h

  5) from t=0 to t=4 h

- the change of concentration between the levels 0 and 5 is accomplished within 0.1 h.

The results of the computer calculation together with empirical values from Fig.8 are given in Table 5.

Case	1	2	3	4	5
SF cumputed	80	43	24	89	75
SF experiment	88	50	25	90	80

Table 5: Computed and experimental values of the surviving fraction

Example 2

This is a computer simulation of the double-labelling experiment reported by Fietkau et al. (see Section 2). The use of the program CELLU gives the possibility of accounting for cell division, which is neglected in the model of Fig.4, and hence to extend the calculation beyond the period of 16 h, after which the mitotic index rises again.

The following data are reported in the paper by Fietkau et al. (1984):

- T_{G_1} = 4, T_S = 10, T_{G_2+M} = 1 (ascites tumor L 1210)
- PF = 1
- a single dose of ara-C (200 mg/kg) is injected at t=0
- 87% of cells in S and 21% of cells in G_1 at time of injection are killed

The ascites tumor L 1210 has a distribution of cycle times with very small variance. Furthermore, there is a short interval of 1/2 h between C^{14}-labelling and injection of ara-C. Therefore, we have decided to represent the cell cycle by 30 compartments of 1/2 h duration, 8 for G_1, 20 for S and 1 for each G_2 and M. The FLM curve generated by this model has already been shown in Fig. 10 of Chapter II. Since PF=1, the division factor α is 2.

At first, the stable age distribution of this model is computed, using the program MITO or CELLU itself. The development of the differently labelled subpopulations will be simulated separately by choosing the appropriate initial values for the x_i (i=1,...,30), namely the values of the stable age distribution for the compartments occupied by the subpopulation and zeroes for the rest. For example, the calculation for the purely H^3-labelled cells starts with the initial values

        4.57, 4.46, 4.36, 0, ..., 0, 2.34

The main results of the computation are shown in Fig.11. It turns out that the relative size of the 4 subpopulations of interphases rises and falls in a similar way as in the experiment (see Fig.3), but with different extent. The rise of the fraction of purely H^3-labelled cells is much less dramatic, while the unlabelled cells attain a level of about 40%.

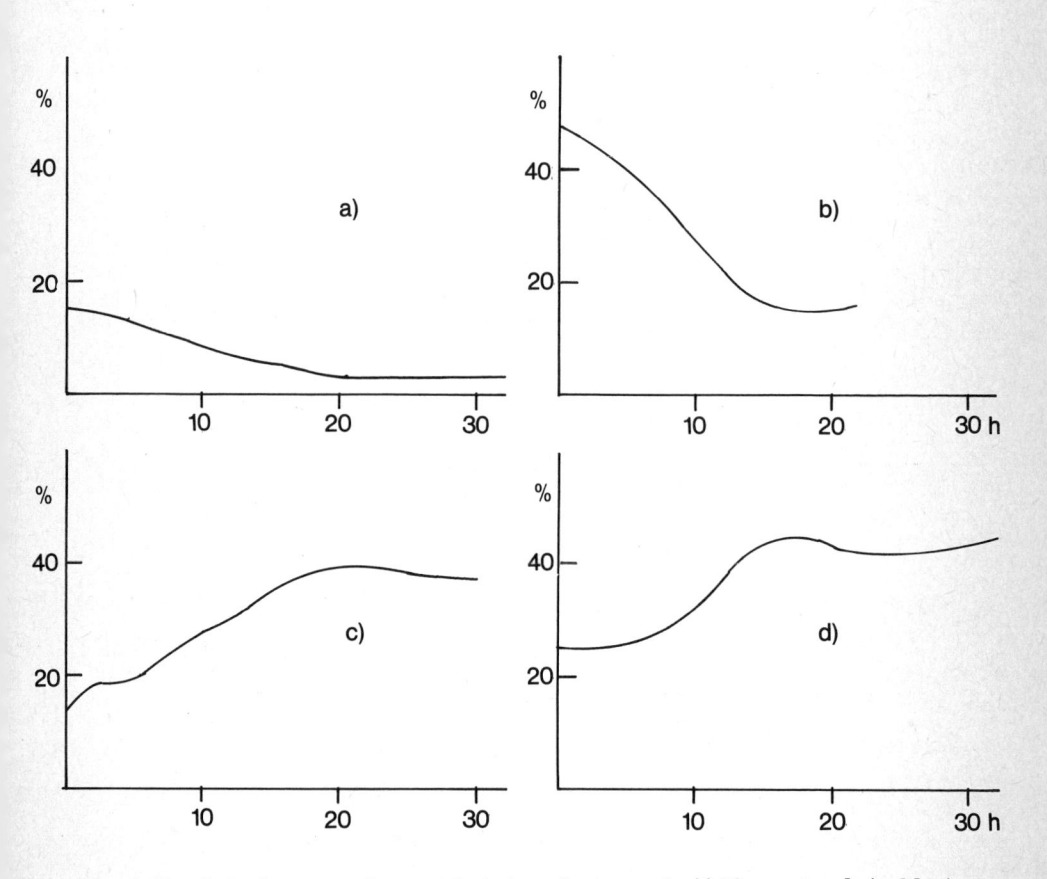

Fig.11: Calculated percentage of interphases of differenty labelled subpopulations as a function of time after ara-C. a) purely C^{14}-labelled, b) double labelled, c) H^3-labelled, d) unlabelled

6. Implications for drug testing

Before a new drug can be used in cancer therapy, it must be tested
under various experimental conditions. At first, the effect on tumor
cell lines in vitro is examined. The dependence of cell survival on
concentration and exposure time, phase-specific cell kill, and retardation of the cell cycle during and after treatment can be measured
in vitro, using colony assays, synchronization and labelling experiments. However, those cytokinetic drug effects which are related to
the distinction of proliferating and resting cells, must be studied
in vivo.

If the agent has exhibited cytotoxic properties in vitro, then it
passes to the next stage, where its effect on transplanted or auto-
chthonous tumors in animals and the possibility of curing these animals with adequate doses of the agent is tested. Since single dose
testing has become obsolete, a schedule for sequential doses has to
be chosen. Gray (1983) has pointed out that potentially effective
drugs may be rejected, when randomly selected schedules of administration are used in testing. This is illustrated by a model calculation, where the effect of ara-C on stem cells of the intestinal epithelium (crypt cells) and on a slow-growing mammary tumor of the mouse
for various periodicities of administration is compared. Under the
assumption that reduction of the crypt cells by 3 orders of magnitude
results in death, whereas reduction of the tumor by 9 orders of magnitude results in cure, Gray has calculated the time to kill, T_k, and
the time to cure, T_{cu}. It results, that both T_k and T_{cu} depend on the
periodicity p, such that $T_k < T_{cu}$ for $p < 14h$ and $T_k > T_{cu}$ for $p \geq 14h$,
i.e. cure is possible, but only for $p \geq 14h$.

The size of a cell population under periodic treatment with a cytotoxic drug is described by a function of the form $\pi(t)e^{-Kt}$, where
$K > 0$ and $\pi(t)$ is a positive periodic function (see Sec.2 of the Appendix). The constant K is the quantity of major interest and will be
called the mean decay rate. The assumptions of Gray can be written

$$KT_k = 9 \log 10 \qquad \text{(tumor)}$$
$$KT_{cu} = 3 \log 10 \qquad \text{(crypt)}$$

and therefore the condition $T_k > T_{cu}$ is satisfied, if and only if the
ratio of the decay rate of the tumor and of the crypts is > 3. This
ratio can be used as an index of the therapeutic value of the drug
schedule.

Gray's statement that this therapeutic value depends on the periodicity p, has suggested to attmept a verification with our computer program FLOQ. The phase durations and the division factor of the tumor
(crypts) were assumed to be $G_1 = 17(6)$, $S = 12(5)$, $G_2 + M = 4(1)$, and $\alpha = 1.2$
(1.5). A division factor $\alpha = 1.5$ in a normal renewal tissue is justified
by the recovery process after each dose. We assumed cell kill in S-
phase, but no retardation of the cell cycle. The results are shown
in Table 6.

Period	K_1	K_2	$K_1 : K_2$
10 h	.0378 h^{-1}	.01315 h^{-1}	2.87
12	.0363	.00838	4.33
14	.0341	.00739	4.61
16	.0316	.00733	4.31
18	.0289	.00636	4.54

Table 6: Computed decay rates under periodic treatment
of tumor (K_1) and intestinal crypts (K_2)

The ratio $K_1 : K_2$ jumps from 2.87 to 4.33, when p increases from 10 to
12h, and then remains nearly at the same level. With the assumptions

of Gray this means that cure is possible with p ≥ 12h. The difference
between this and Gray's result may be explained by our assumption
that the cell cycle is not retarded by the drug.

The recruitment of resting cells is another factor which requires a
careful choice of the time schedule in drug testing. Toxicity to the
normal renewal tissues is highly schedule-dependent, if a great fraction of the stem cells is resting under normal conditions. This fact,
which has been observed years ago in the clinic (Frei et al.,1969),
should be taken into account in drug testing, too. An experimental
framework for recruitment studies has been proposed in Section 4.

7. Potential implications for therapy

The crucial problem of cancer chemotherapy is to kill a great number
of cancer cells and to leave enough normal cells alive. The normal
cell populations, which are in danger during cytostatic treatment, are
the renewal tissues: the hemopoietic system, the mucosa of the gastrointestinal tract, and the skin. In these tissues cell loss is equal
to cell production under normal conditions, and therefore they are
in a steady state. But there is a reserve of resting stem cells, which
are stimulated to proliferation after abnormal cell loss and allow
the tissue to grow and to recover from depletion. However, the number
of proliferating cells is reduced and growth is stopped, as soon as
the normal level is attained again.

It is the goal of curative chemotherapy to reduce the number of tumor
cells to a level, where the immune defense of the patient is capable
of doing the rest. This requires that the hemopoietic system is left

in a good state. Usually a chemotherapeutic treatment is subdivided into the phases of induction, consolidation and maintainance. During induction cycle-unspecific agents, i.e. agents that kill resting as well as cycling cells, are used, because the proliferative fraction of the tumor is small. Although a remission (this means, in rough terms, a 100- to 1000-fold decrease of the tumor and disappearance of symptoms) may be achieved at the end of induction, the treatment must be continued, in order to destroy the remaining tumor cell population which attempts to resume exponential growth with a high proliferative fraction. In these consolidation and maintainance phases of therapy the patient receives cycle- and phase-specific drugs, which are less toxic, but have a strong effect on rapidly growing tumors. This general rationale for the choice of drugs was applied by Clarkson in the design of his protocol for acute lymphocytic leukemia (Clarkson, 1974).

Each phase of treatment consists of several 'courses' and a course consists of an active period τ_A, during which a cytotoxic agent is administered n times with periodicity p, followed by a rest period τ_R. Instead of a single drug a combination may be applied, each drug with a different periodicity. During τ_A the size of the tumor and of the normal tissues is reduced, and during τ_R it increases with different velocities. In the following we refer only to the tumor and to the normal hemopoietic stem cells. The clinician would prefer to study changes in the populations of mature cells in the peripheral blood, but for a basic discussion of the recovery process it is necessary to consider first of all a model for the depression and recovery of the stem cell pool in the bone marrow.

Let us suppose that in each course the rest period τ_R is long enough for full recovery of the normal bone marrow, and let R_i be the time necessary to recover from cell loss during the i-th course. We also define a recovery time R_i' for the tumor, namely the time necessary to regrow to the size before the active period of course i. Now, if $R_i < R_i'$ (i=1,2,...) and if in each course τ_R is chosen between R_i and R_i', then the tumor size is reduced step by step, while the normal bone marrow achieves complete recovery during the rest period of each course (Fig.12).

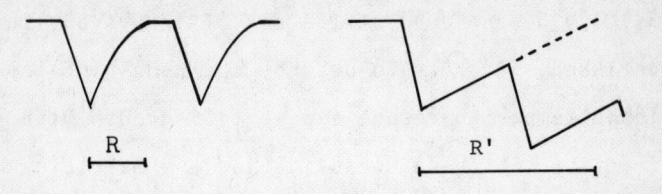

Fig.12. Different response of normal renewal tissue (left) and
tumor (right) to repeated courses of treatment.

This consideration is a current issue in clinical oncology, but there are still several open questions related with it. Can R_i and R_i' actually be determined? What shall be done if $R_i > R_i'$? Is it possible to increase $R_i' - R_i$ by a change in p, n, or the single dose?

As to the bone marrow, the answer to the first question is negative. The time delay between loss of stem cells and the related symptoms in the peripheral blood as well as the difficulty of sampling stem cells from the bone marrow are the reasons. The rest period can be adapted to the recovery time of the normal bone marrow only after several courses of treatment, if necessary. As to the tumor, it may be possible to determine the recovery time during the induction phase, when the tumor burden is great enough to be accessible to measurement. During consolidation and maintainance the recovery time of the tumor cannot be measured directly with methods available today, but it can be calculated provided that there is enough information on drug sensitivity and growth kinetics of the rest tumor.

It is obvious that the recovery time depends on the fraction of surviving cells which are left after an active period, and on the growth rate during the rest period. The surviving fraction after τ_A depends on the mean decay rate K defined in the preceding section, namely SF= $\exp(-K\tau_A)$. If, during the rest period, the tumor is growing exponentially with rate ρ, then the recovery time is R=Kτ_A/ρ. But today we have no data on drug response and growth kinetics of tumors after several weeks or months of treatment and we do not know whether we can extrapolate from parameters measured before or during early stages of treatment (Gray, 1983).

The answer to the 3rd question is positive in the sense, that $R_i - R_i'$ depends on p, if the cytotoxic agent is phase-specific and if the tumor and the hemopoietic stem cells have different cell cycle parameters. For S-phase specific drugs it has already been suggested by many authors that the most effective interval between doses is $p_{max}=T_S$. Furthermore the model with uniform cycle time predicts that the less effective interval is $p_{min}=T_C$. Of course p_{max} and p_{min} are increased to some extent which depends on the single dose, if the agent induces also a retardation of the G_1 phase.

These intuitive considerations have been checked by calculations with the computer program FLOQ (see Sec.5), which is based on the cytokinetic model of Takahashi (see Chap.I). This model, which consists of a system of linear differential equations, cannot describe populations with a Gompertz growth curve, but this doesn't matter so much, since phase-specific agents are applied mainly during consolidation and maintainance therapy, i.e. when the tumor is thrown back to an early stage with exponential growth. In the calculations it was assumed that an S-phase specific agent was applied with periodicities p between 6 and 36 h to a tumor A with T_S = 8h, T_C = 16h, α = 1.2 and to a tumor B with T_S = 12h, T_C = 24h, α = 1.31. The different values of the division factor were chosen such that the growth rate was approximately

equal in spite of different cycle times. The FLM curve of tumor A
(see Fig.13) shows that the variation of the cycle time corresponds
to that observed in human tumors. The single dose was proportional
to p, such that the dose applied per day was equal in all cases. The
concentration of the drug in the tumor was proportional to the single
dose and decayed with a half life $T_{1/2}$ = 1 h.

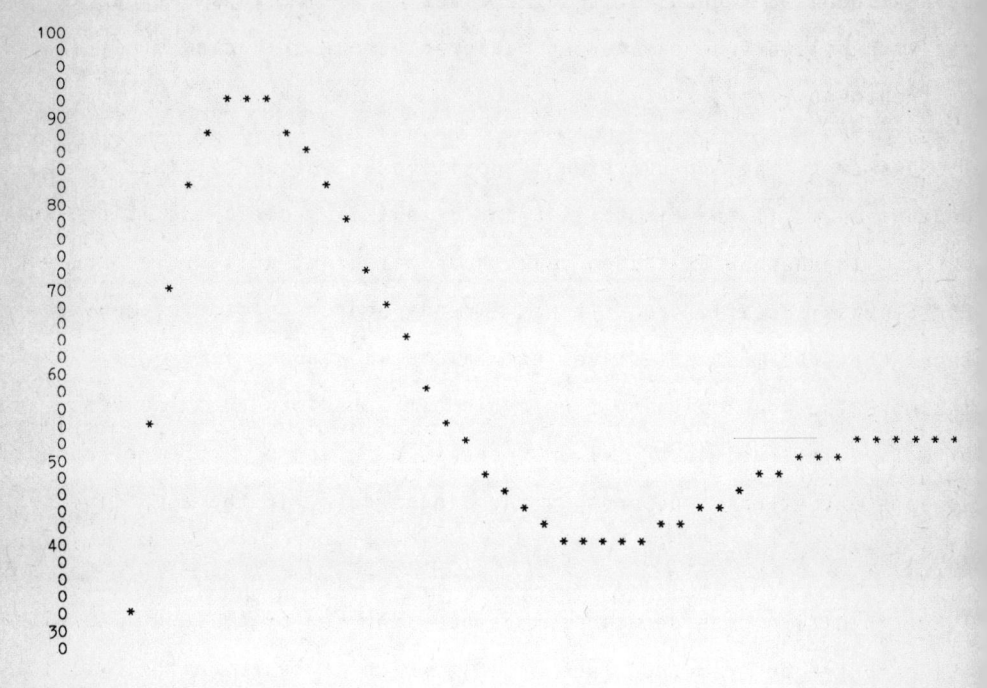

Fig.13. Calculated FLM curve of tumor A. The FLM curve of
         tumor B is similar.

The results are shown in Table 7. It is seen, that neither p_{max} = T_S
nor p_{min} = T_C is satisfied. Both decay rates are decreasing functions
of p. But the difference between decay rates exhibits a maximum at
p=14 and a minimum at p=24. So the original statement about the role
of T_S and T_C (12h resp. 24h for B) is saved in a broader sense. Similar comparisons can be made between a tumor and normal bone marrow,
and it will become evident that the difference in decay rates and hence

the difference in recovery times depends on p.

period		6	8	10	12	14	16	18
decay rate	A	.434	.430	.410	.374	.332	.299	.281
	B	.419	.419	.411	.394	.369	.335	.294
difference		.015	.011	-.001	-.020	-.037	-.036	-.013

period		20	22	24	28	32	36
decay rate	A	.271	.263	.252	.222	.194	.172
	B	.254	.223	.201	.176	.162	.146
difference		.017	.040	.051	.046	.032	.026

Table 7. Comparison of mean decay rates of model tumors
A and B under periodic treatment. Decay rates
multiplied with 10.

The effect of variation of the periodicity has been stressed also by
the work of Dibrov et al. (1985). The treatment of acute myeloblastic
leukemia with an S-phase specific drug and a periodic schedule was
examined by Rubinow and Lebowitz (1976b), using a mathematical model
that includes growth regulation for the normal bone marrow (Rubinow
and Lebowitz, 1976a). They assumed that a dose that kills 90% of cells
in S, whether leukemic or normal, was administered n=10 times with periodicity p=15, 18, 20, and 24 h, and that the active period of length
(n-1)p was followed by a rest period of three weeks. It turned out
that with p=15 both normal and leukemic cells were eliminated with
equal fractions at the long term, while at p=18, 20, and 24 h the normal population achieved recovery but the leukemic population decreased
from course to course, most rapidly at p=20 h. They relate this result
to the length of S, which is about 15 h in normal bone marrow and 20 h
in leukemic myeloblasts.

The attempt to establish an optimal period is quite different from another cytokinetic approach in cancer therapy, which has been called synchronization therapy (Klein and Lennartz, 1974). There, a blocking agent (vincristine) should generate a synchronous wave of cells and then an "executive" phase-specific drug should be administered exactly at the moment, when the maximal number of cells is in the sensitive phase. But later it was shown that the cells supposed to be reversibly blocked in mitosis were in fact doomed to die or to produce sterile daughter cells (Camplejohn, 1980). Therefore, if patients were cured with this treatment modality, it was due to the cell kill capacity of both agents. Furthermore, even with an ideal blocking agent a reasonable degree of synchronization in vivo can be obtained only if the concentration of the agent falls rapidly to zero after a period of continuous infusion.

It is useful to remark that phase-specific cell kill induces a certain degree of synchrony, since nearly all cells in the sensitive phase are taken away. Periodic treatment with a phase-specific agent is therefore a sort of synchronization therapy where the executive drug is also the synchronizing drug. Recruitment of resting cells must also be considered. If many cells are recruited during a short time, then a synchronous wave enters the S-phase and after that the labelling index attains a maximum. Applying the next dose at the moment of the maximum produces the greatest cell kill. An attempt to exploit this fact in therapy was made by Smets et al. (1982).

The work of Rubinow and Lebowitz, the approach of Smets et al. and our own calculations stress the point that the usual intervals of drug administration 8, 12, 24 hr etc., which are chosen for purely technical reasons, may be wrong in cancer therapy. "Odd" intervals, such as 20h, may be more effective against the tumor and less toxic for the bone marrow. If it were possible to determine phase durations and other kinetic parameters of normal and tumor cells in the patient during therapy - and we should assume that it will be possible in the future - then the optimal periodicity p could be determined with the help of an appropriate mathematical model and computer experiments.

APPENDIX

1. Limit theorems for matrix models

In this section the behavior of the Takahashi model for $t \to \infty$ is investigated with the aid of the classical theory of Frobenius on non-negative irreducible matrices. The reader should be familiar with the basic concepts of matrix algebra, such as matrix, vector, sum and product of matrices, product of a matrix and a vector, product of a vector and a complex number. We will consider only real n-dimensional square matrices and n-dimensional vectors. The identity matrix will be denoted with I, the zero matrix and the zero vector with 0.

A real or complex number λ is called an eigenvalue of the matrix A if there is a vector $V \neq 0$ (called eigenvector) such that $AV = \lambda V$. The eigenvalues are the roots of the n-th degree algebraic equation $\det(A - \lambda I) = 0$.

If $AV = \lambda V$ and s is a real number then $(A+sI)V = AV + sV = (\lambda + s)V$, hence $\lambda + s$ is an eigenvalue and V an eigenvector of the matrix A+sI.

A matrix A with elements a_{ik} $(i,k=1,\ldots,n)$ is called nonnegative, $A \geq 0$, if all its elements are nonnegative. In the same way, positive matrices as well as nonnegative and positive vectors are defined. If A and B are matrices (vectors), then $A \geq B$ means that $A-B \geq 0$.

With any matrix $A \geq 0$ is associated a graph consisting of n points $P_1, \ldots, P_n$ and at most n^2 arrows, such that there is an arrow from P_i to P_k, if and only if $a_{ik} > 0$. A is called reducible if the set

$\{P_1,\ldots,P_n\}$ splits into two subsets S_1 and S_2, such that $a_{ik}=0$ whenever $P_k \in S_1$, $P_i \in S_2$. By renumbering the points we can achieve the separation $S_1 = \{P_1,\ldots,P_m\}$, $S_2 = \{P_{m+1},\ldots,P_n\}$. If rows and columns of A are renumbered in the same way, then A takes the form

$$A = \begin{pmatrix} A_1 & B_1 \\ 0 & A_2 \end{pmatrix} \qquad\qquad (1.1)$$

with square sumbatrices A_1 (m rows) and A_2 (n-m rows) and a lower left submatrix containing only zeroes. If A cannot be reduced to this form by renumbering rows and columns, then it is called irreducible. Examples of irreducible and reducible matrices are (respectively)

$$A = \begin{pmatrix} 0 & 0 & 1 \\ 1 & 0 & 0 \\ 0 & 1 & 0 \end{pmatrix} \qquad\qquad B = \begin{pmatrix} 0 & 1 & 1 \\ 1 & 0 & 1 \\ 0 & 0 & 1 \end{pmatrix}.$$

The associated graphs are shown in Fig.1. In graph b) there is a separation of the set $\{P_1,P_2,P_3\}$ into the subsets $S_1=\{P_1,P_2\}$ and $S_2=\{P_3\}$.

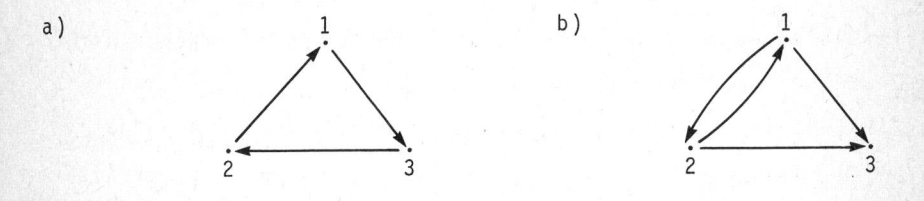

a)

b)

Fig.1: Graphs of matrices
a) irreducible
b) reducible

The following criterion of irreducibility will be useful:

The matrix A is irreducible if for any pair (i,k) there is a one-way route (a sequence of equally directed arrows) from P_i to P_k in the associated graph.

In order to prove the criterion we assume that a one-way route between any two points exists, and consider a partition of the set $\{P_1,\ldots,P_n\}$ into 2 nonvoid subsets S_1 and S_2. If $P_k \in S_1$, $P_i \in S_2$ then there is an one-way route from P_i to P_k which contains a point $P_{i'}$ (the last in S_2) and a point $P_{k'}$ (the first in S_1) such that $a_{i'k'} > 0$. This is true for any partition, and therefore A cannot be reduced to the form given in (1.1), i.e. A is irreducible.

A nonnegative matrix with positive elements in the subdiagonal and the right upper corner is irreducible. Indeed, in the graph of such a matrix there is an arrow from P_i to P_{i+1} (i=1,...,n-1) and from P_n to P_1.

The eigenvalues of nonnegative irreducible matrices have been investigated by Frobenius. His main results will be stated now.

<u>Theorem 1</u> (Frobenius 1912): (1) An irreducible nonnegative matrix A has a positive eigenvalue r which is greater or equal than the absolute value of any other eigenvalue. To r belongs a positive eigenvector, and no other eigenvalue has this property.
(2) If A has k eigenvalues of absolute value r then A has the form, after suitable renumbering of rows and columns,

$$
A = \begin{pmatrix}
0 & 0 & 0 & \cdots\cdots & 0 & A_k \\
A_1 & 0 & 0 & \cdots\cdots & 0 & 0 \\
0 & A_2 & 0 & \cdots\cdots & 0 & 0 \\
\cdot & \cdot & \cdot & \cdots\cdots & \cdot & \cdot \\
0 & \cdot & \cdot & \cdots\ 0 & A_{k-1} & 0
\end{pmatrix}
$$

with square submatrices $A_1,\ldots,A_k$ in the subdiagonal and the right upper corner.

For the sake of simplicity we have announced only the statements necessary for the purpose of population kinetics. A complete version and a simple proof of the theorem are found in a paper by Wielandt (1949).
A direct consequence of Theorem 1 is the fact that the positive eigenvalue r is strictly greater than the real part of any other eigenvalue.

Now consider the matrix

$$M = \begin{pmatrix} -b_1 & 0 & 0 & \cdots\cdots\cdots & \alpha a_n \\ a_1 & -b_2 & 0 & \cdots\cdots\cdots & 0 \\ 0 & a_2 & -b_3 & \cdots\cdots\cdots & 0 \\ \cdot & \cdot & \cdot & \cdots\cdots\cdots & \cdot \\ 0 & \cdot & \cdot & \cdots 0 \quad a_{n-1} & -b_n \end{pmatrix} \tag{1.2}$$

where $a_i, b_i > 0$ $(i=1,\ldots,n)$, $\alpha > 0$. On adding a suitable positive s to the diagonal elements, we can get a nonnegative matrix which is irreducible. Therefore M has a real eigenvalue ρ, which may be negative but in any case is greater than the real part of any other eigenvalue. To ρ belongs a positive eigenvector V_o.

The system of differential equations (7.5, Chap.I) which builds up the Takahashi model may be written in matrix form:

$$dX/dt = MX \tag{1.3}$$

If all the eigenvalues of M are simple, then eq. (3) has the general solution

$$X(t) = c_0 e^{\rho t} V_0 + \sum_{i=1}^{n-1} c_i e^{\lambda_i t} V_i$$

where the λ_i are eigenvalues with real part less than ρ, the V_i are eigenvectors and the c_i are constants that depend on the initial values. Since $\rho > Re(\lambda_i)$ we have

$$\lim_{t \to \infty} X(t)e^{-\rho t} = c_0 V_0 \qquad (1.4)$$

The next theorem tells us, how c_0 can be calculated from the initial values.

Theorem 2: Suppose that $V_0 = (\sigma_1, \ldots, \sigma_n)$ is the positive eigenvector belonging to ρ. Let the positive numbers $\varepsilon_1, \ldots, \varepsilon_n$ be defined by the relations

$$\varepsilon_{i+1} = \frac{\rho + b_i}{a_i} \varepsilon_i \qquad (i=1, \ldots, n-1) \qquad (1.5)$$

$$\sum_{i=1}^{n} \sigma_i \varepsilon_i = 1 \qquad (1.6)$$

Then the solution of (3) with the initial condition $X(0) = (\xi_1, \ldots, \xi_n)$ satisfies eq. (4) with $c_0 = \sum_{i=1}^{n} \varepsilon_i \xi_i$.

Proof: Since the set of eigenvectors is linearly independent, the i-th unit vector $E_i = (0, \ldots, 0, 1, 0, \ldots, 0)$ has a unique representation

$$E_i = \varepsilon_i V_0 + c_i^1 V_1 + \ldots + c_i^{n-1} V_{n-1} \qquad (1.7)$$

where ε_i is not yet specified.

For i=1,...,n-1 the matrix $M_i = M+b_iI$ satisfies

$$M_iE_i = a_iE_{i+1}$$

$$M_iV_0 = (\rho+b_i)V_0$$

$$M_iV_k = (\lambda_k+b_i)V_k \qquad k=1,...,n-1$$

Multiplying eq. (7) with M_i we have

$$M_iE_i = \varepsilon_i(\rho+b_i)V_0 + c_i^1(\lambda_1+b_i)V_1 + \ldots \qquad (i=1,...,n-1)$$

and hence

$$E_{i+1} = \frac{\rho+b_i}{a_i} \varepsilon_iV_0 + \ldots$$

Therefore the uniqueness of the representation (7) implies (5). Multiplying eq. (7) with σ_i and taking the sum from 1 to n we obtain

$$V_0 = \sum\sigma_iE_i$$

$$= (\sum \sigma_i\varepsilon_i)V_0 + \ldots$$

and hence eq. (6).

Now the solution of the differential equation (3) with the initial condition $X(0) = E_i$ satisfies $\lim\limits_{t \to \infty} X(t)e^{-\rho t} = \varepsilon_iV_0$. Since the solution of a linear differential equation depends linearly on the initial condition $X(0) = \sum\xi_iE_i$ the proof is complete.

Theorem 2 gives us the possibility of calculating the future size of an initially synchronized cell population without solving the system of differential equations (7.5) explicitly.

An application refers to the final level of the index of pulse labelling. If an asynchronous cell population is labelled by a short exposure to H^3-Thymidine then a synchronized subpopulation of labelled cells is produced. At the beginning the labelling index LI has the value $PF \cdot k_S(T_S/T_C)$, where k_S is the correction factor due to the exponential age distribution (see Chapter II). We remember that k_S depends on the position of the S-phase in the cell cycle. Nevertheless the final level of the LI is exactly T_S/T_C. In the proof of this statement we will assume that there is no alteration of the cell cycle by labelling.

Theorem 3: Suppose that the proliferating part of a cell population can be described by eq. (3) and that $a_i = a_{i+1}$ and $b_i = b_{i+1}$ ($i=1,\ldots,n-1$). If the population has the stable age distribution then the fraction of labelled cells among the proliferating cells after pulse labelling tends to the limit T_S/T_C.

Remark: The statement that the LI also tends to T_S/T_C is a consequence of this theorem and is proved in Sec.1, Chap.II.

Proof: From the eigenvalue equation $MV_o = \rho V_o$ we deduce that the components of V_o satisfy

$$\sigma_{i+1} = \frac{a_i}{\rho + b_{i+1}} \, \sigma_i \qquad (i=1,\ldots,n-1)$$

From this and eq. (5) we obtain

$$\sigma_{i+1}\varepsilon_{i+1} = \frac{\rho + b_i}{\rho + b_{i+1}} \, \sigma_i \varepsilon_i \qquad (i=1,\ldots,n-1)$$

Therefore the assumption $b_i = b_{i+1}$ and eq. (6) imply

$$\sigma_i \varepsilon_i = 1/n \qquad (i=1,\ldots,n)$$

Denote the age distribution of all P-cells with $X(t)$ and that of the labelled P-cells with $Y(t)$ and suppose that the S-phase is represented by m and G_1 by k compartments. The initial conditions are

$$X(0) = zV_o$$

$$Y(0) = z(0,\ldots,0,\sigma_{k+1},\ldots,\sigma_{k+m},0,\ldots,0)$$

where z is a positive number. Then the preceding theorem implies

$$\lim_{t \to \infty} X(t)e^{-\rho t} = zV_o$$

$$\lim_{t \to \infty} Y(t)e^{-\rho t} = z \sum_{i=k+1}^{k+m} \sigma_i \varepsilon_i V_o = z \frac{m}{n} V_o$$

Thus the labelled subpopulation is by a factor m/n smaller, i.e. with the terminology of Chapter II

$$\lim_{t \to \infty} \frac{P^*(t)}{P(t)} = \frac{m}{n}$$

Equation (3) is essentially the Takahashi model (7.5, Chap.I) with passage rates a_i. The difference $b_i - a_i$, if it is positive, expresses cell death at stage i. We know already that a stage with passage rate a and loss rate λ has a mean duration $(a+\lambda)^{-1}$ and that the mean duration of a phase is the sum of the duration of its stages. Therefore the assumptions $a_{i+1} = a_i$, $b_{i+1} = b_i$ (i=1,...,n-1) imply $T_S/T_C = m/n$ and

$$\lim_{t \to \infty} \frac{P^*(t)}{P(t)} = \frac{T_S}{T_C} \tag{1.8}$$

Another application of Theorem 2 refers to the extended model of tumor growth (Chap.I). Let

$$X(t) = \begin{pmatrix} P(t) \\ Q(t) \end{pmatrix} \qquad M = \begin{pmatrix} a_{11} & a_{12} \\ a_{21} & a_{22} \end{pmatrix} = \begin{pmatrix} -b_1 & \alpha a_2 \\ a_1 & -b_2 \end{pmatrix}$$

and $V_0 = (1,r)$. Applying eq. (5) and (6) and eq. (4.6) of Chap.I we obtain $\varepsilon_2 = a_{12}r\varepsilon_1/a_{21}$ and $\varepsilon_1 + r\varepsilon_2 = 1$, hence

$$\varepsilon_1 = \frac{a_{21}}{a_{21} + a_{12}r^2} \qquad\qquad \varepsilon_2 = \frac{a_{12}r}{a_{21} + a_{12}r^2} \qquad (1.9)$$

Therefore, eq. (4.8) of Chap.I follows if Theorem 2 is applied with $\xi_1 = P_0$, $\xi_2 = Q_0$, and $c_0 = c(P_0, Q_0)$.

2. A model with periodic parameters

If cell kinetic parameters undergo periodic change as in cell populations exhibiting diurnal rhythms or perturbed by periodic applications of cytotoxic drugs, then the constant coefficients in the equations of the Takahashi model must be replaced by periodic coefficients. Therefore we consider now the system

$$X' = A(t)X \qquad\qquad (2.1)$$

where A is periodic with period ω, i.e.

$$A(t+\omega) = A(t) \quad \text{for all } t. \qquad\qquad (2.2)$$

The properties of solutions of eq. (1) are revealed by the theory of Floquet (see e.g. Coddington and Levinson, Theory of Ordinary Differential Equations, 1955). The use of this theory and of the theorem of Frobenius in the treatment of diurnal rhythms has been proposed by Klein and Valleron (1977). According to Floquet each solution of eq. (1) has the form

$$X(t) = \sum_{i=0}^{n-1} c_i e^{\lambda_i t} V_i(t) \qquad (2.3)$$

where the c_i are constants and the V_i are periodic vectors with period ω. Furthermore, if the system (1) is a model of a proliferating cell population similar to the Takahashi model, then one of the λ_i, say λ_0 is real and

$$\lim_{t \to \infty} X(t)e^{-\lambda_0 t} = c_0 V_0(t) \qquad (2.4)$$

A rigorous proof of this fact is missing in the paper by Klein and Valleron and will be given now.

First we explain how the λ_i in eq. (3) are obtained. Let $\Phi(t)$ be a fundamental matrix (i.e. a matrix whose columns are n linearly independent solutions of eq. (1)) and let μ_i (i=0,...,n-1) be the eigenvalues of the constant matrix $C := \Phi(\omega)\Phi(0)^{-1}$, the so called monodromy matrix. Then $\lambda_i = \frac{1}{\omega} \log \mu_i$. The μ_i and hence the λ_i do not depend on the choice of the fundamental matrix, therefore we may choose $\Phi(0)=I$. Since the columns of $\Phi(\omega)$ are linearly independent, all the μ_i are $\neq 0$. If C has multiple eigenvalues then some terms of the sum in eq. (3) are multiplied by a power of t.

We must show that one of the λ_i is real and strictly greater than the real parts of the rest. Since $\mu_0 > |\mu_1|$ implies $\log \mu_0 > \log|\mu_1| = Re(\log \mu_1) = \omega Re\lambda_1$ and vice versa, it is necessary and sufficient to show that one of the μ_i is positive and strictly greater than the absolute values of the rest. For this purpose we will prove that $C = \Phi(\omega) > 0$ (all elements are positive) and then apply the 2nd part of Theorem 1. In doing so we will use the following theorem, which is stated without proof.

Theorem 4 (Wielandt, 1949): Let B be a nonnegative irreducible matrix and Y a nonnegative vector, $Y \neq 0$. Then the vector $(I+B)^{n-1}Y$ is positive.

Concerning the periodic matrix $A(t)$, we need some additional assumptions which are justified by its biological meaning. It is reasonable to assume that the flow of cells is never reversed and not completely blocked all the time. The 1st assumption implies that

$$a_{ik}(t) \geq 0 \qquad \text{for } i \neq k, \text{ for all } t. \qquad (2.5)$$

A stronger form of the 2nd assumption says that there is a time interval (t_1, t_2) during which there is no complete block at any stage of the cell cycle. This means that there is a nonnegative matrix G with positive elements in the subdiagonal and the right upper corner such that

$$a_{ik}(t) \geq g_{ik} \qquad \text{for } i \neq k \quad \text{and} \quad t_1 \leq t \leq t_2. \qquad (2.6)$$

Note that G is irreducible.

Now let $X(t)$ be a solution of eq. (1) with $X(0) \geq 0$ and $\neq 0$. The proof that $X(t) \geq 0$ for $t > 0$ is obtained easily with the aid of a perturbation technique and is omitted here. Instead we will prove that $X(\omega) > 0$ which implies $\Phi(\omega) > 0$.

Let $\gamma > 0$ be such that $A(t) \geq - \gamma I$ $(0 \leq t \leq \omega)$. Then, using ineq. (6), we obtain

$$A(t)X(t) \geq (G - \gamma I)X(t) \qquad (t_1 \leq t \leq t_2).$$

If an approximate solution X_h is computed with the Euler method with step width $h < \gamma^{-1}$ then

$$X_h(t+h) - X_h(t) = hA(t)X_h(t)$$

$$X_h(t+h) = (1+hA(t))X_h(t)$$

$$\geq \{(1-h\gamma)I + hG\}X_h(t)$$

$$\geq (1-h\gamma)\{I+B\}X_h(t) \qquad\qquad (t_1 \leq t \leq t_2)$$

where $B=hG$ is nonnegative and irreducible.

Applying Theorem 4 to B and to the vector $X(t_1)$ we obtain

$$(I+B)^{n-1}X(t_1) > 0.$$

Now we choose h such that $m = (t_2-t_1)/h$ is integer and greater than n-1. Then by induction

$$X_h(t_2) = X_h(t_1+mh)$$

$$\geq (1-h\gamma)^m(I+B)^mX(t_1) > 0.$$

For some integer p let $h'=h/p$. Since $B \geq 0$ we have $(I+\frac{1}{p}B)^p \geq I+B$ and hence

$$X_{h'}(t_2) \geq (1-h'\gamma)^{pm}(I+\frac{1}{p}B)^{pm}X(t_1)$$

$$\geq (1-h'\gamma)^{pm}(I+B)^mX(t_1).$$

If $p \to \infty$ then $h' \to 0$ and hence the exact solution satisfies

$$X(t_2) \geq e^{-\gamma(t_2-t_1)}(I+B)^mX(t_1) > 0.$$

From the i-th equation of system (1) it follows that

$$x_i'(t) \geq a_{ii}(t)x_i(t) \geq -\gamma x_i(t)$$

$$x_i(\omega) \geq x_i(t)e^{-\gamma(\omega-t)} \qquad\qquad (t \leq \omega).$$

Therefore, if X is positive in $t=t_2$ then it is so in $t=\omega$. Since this is true for each column of the fundamental matrix $\Phi(t)$, we see that $\Phi(\omega) > 0$. Hence $\Phi(\omega)$ is irreducible and has a positive eigenvalue r. Furthermore, it does not satisfy the condition of the 2nd part of Theorem 1, and therefore the absolute value of all the other eigenvalues is strictly less than r. So we have obtained the following

Theorem 5: Suppose that conditions (5) and (6) are satisfied, and let Φ be the fundamental matrix for eq. (1) with $\Phi(0)=I$. Then $\Phi(\omega)$ has a unique positive eigenvalue r, and any solution of eq. (1) satisfies

$$\lim_{t \to \infty} X(t)e^{-\rho t} = V(t) \tag{2.7}$$

where $\rho = \frac{1}{\omega} \log r$ and $V(t)$ is a periodic vector with period ω.

Applied to cell kinetics, this theorem implies that the growth pattern of cell populations with periodic perturbations is very similar to that considered before. The only difference between (2.7) and (1.4) is the periodicity of the vector V. The growth parameter ρ can be calculated by the computer program FLOQ (see Sec.5, Chap.III).

3. Pharmacokinetics and the dose-effect relation

In Sec.1 of Chap.III where we have derived a relation between the dose and the fraction of surviving cells, we assumed that the area under the concentration curve

$$AUC = \int_0^\infty C(t) \, dt$$

is proportional to the dose. Now we will give this statement a precise meaning and a rigorous proof.

<u>Theorem 6</u>: Consider a system of n pharmacokinetic compartments K_i with concentration C_i ($i=1,\ldots,n$) and suppose that the C_i satisfy the limit relations

$$C_i(t) \to 0 \quad \text{as} \quad t \to \infty \qquad (i=1,\ldots,n) \qquad (3.1)$$

and the system of differential equations

$$C_i' = \sum_{k=1}^{n} a_{ik} C_k \qquad (i=1,\ldots,n) \qquad (3.2)$$

where $a_{ii} < 0$ and $a_{ik} \geq 0$ for $i \neq k$. If $C_1(0) \neq 0$ and $C_i(0) = 0$ ($i>1$), then the AUC in all compartments is proportional to $C_1(0)$.

Remark: For a bolus application (dose D) into the 1st compartment (volume V_1) we have $C_1(0) = D/V_1$. Hence the theorem states that the AUC in all compartments is proportional to the dose.

<u>Proof:</u> First let's suppose, that the matrix $A = (a_{ik})$ is irreducible. Then the determinant of A is $\neq 0$. For, if det $A = 0$, then there is a vector $X \neq 0$ such that $AX = 0 \cdot X$, i.e. 0 is an eigenvalue of A and X is a constant solution of the differential system $X'=AX$. According to Theorem 1 an eigenvector belonging to 0 could be chosen with non-negative components. But then X would represent a steady state with constant positive concentrations in some compartments, in contradic-

tion to eq. (1).

Integrating the equations of system (2) term by term and using eq. (1), we obtain

$$-C_i(0) = \sum_{i=1}^{n} a_{ik} \int_0^{\infty} C_k(t) \, dt \qquad (3.3)$$

This system of n linear equations in the unknown areas may be written in the condensed form

$$AF = Y \qquad (3.3a)$$

where F is the vector of areas and Y is the vector with components $-C_1(0), 0, \ldots, 0$.

According to Cramer's rule

$$\int_0^{\infty} C_k(t) \, dt = \frac{\det A_k^*}{\det A} \qquad k = 1, \ldots, n$$

where A_k^* is a matrix, whose k-th column contains only one nonzero element: $-C_1(0)$. Therefore $\det A_k^*$ and the area are proportional to $C_1(0)$. When A is reducible, then the rows and columns can be rearranged such that

$$A = \begin{pmatrix} A_1 & B_1 \\ 0 & A_2 \end{pmatrix} \qquad (3.4)$$

where A_1 and A_2 are square submatrices with n_1 resp. n_2 rows. The right side of (3a) has been rearranged too and can be divided into a vector Y_1 of n_1 and Y_2 of n_2 elements. One of the vectors Y_i is zero, the other contains only one non-zero element. With a similar subdivision of the vector F the equation AF = Y can be splitted into the equations

$$A_1F_1 + B_1F_2 = Y_1 \qquad\qquad (3.5a)$$

$$A_2F_2 = Y_2 \qquad\qquad (3.5b)$$

Now suppose, that A_1 and A_2 are irreducible. If $Y_2 = 0$, $Y_1 \neq 0$, then $A_2F_2 = Y_2$ has only the solution $F_2 = 0$, and eq. (5a) reduces to $A_1F_1 = Y_1$. The same argument as before shows that the elements of F_1 are proportional to $C_1(0)$. If $Y_1 = 0$ and $Y_2 \neq 0$, then we deduce at first that the elements of F_2 are proportional to $C_1(0)$, and then that the same holds for F_1, since $A_1F_1 = -B_1F_2$. If one of the matrices A_1 and A_2 or both are reducible, then the subdivision (4) may be applied again and the whole procedure may be repeated until a chain of irreducible matrices along the diagonal of A is found. This is always possible because the n matrices with a_{ii} as unique element are irreducible. This remark completes the proof of Theorem 7.

As an example, we consider a system with three compartments (Fig. 2), which may be gastrointestinal tract (1), blood (2), and tissue (3).

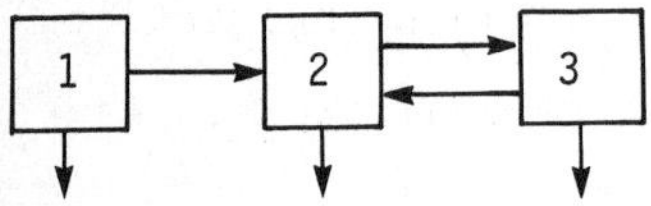

Fig.2: Compartment system

In treating an actual system we prefer to change the sign of the a_{ii} and to reverse the order of the indices of a_{ij}, such that a_{ij} becomes the rate of flow from K_i to K_j. With these conventions we have the differential equations

$$C_2' = -a_{22}C_2 + a_{32}C_3 + a_{12}C_1 \qquad\qquad (3.6a)$$

$$C_3' = a_{23}C_2 - a_{33}C_3 \qquad\qquad (3.6b)$$

$$C_1' = \qquad\qquad - a_{11}C_1 \qquad\qquad (3.6c)$$

The matrix of the system is reducible, but

$$A_1 = \begin{pmatrix} -a_{22} & a_{32} \\ a_{23} & -a_{33} \end{pmatrix}$$

is irreducible. We assume $C_1(0) \neq 0$ and write

$$f_i = \int_0^\infty C_i(t) \, dt$$

From eq. (6c) we obtain $f_1 = C_1(0)/a_{11}$, and from (6a) and (6b)

$$-a_{22}f_2 + a_{32}f_3 = -a_{12}f_1 \qquad (3.7a)$$

$$a_{23}f_2 - a_{33}f_3 = 0 \qquad (3.7b)$$

and hence, using Cramer's rule

$$f_2 = \frac{a_{12}a_{33}}{\det A_1} f_1 \qquad\qquad f_3 = \frac{a_{12}a_{23}}{\det A_1} f_1$$

Therefore the areas f_1, f_2, f_3 are proportional to $C_1(0)$.

List of Symbols

T_C	cycle time (generation time)
T_{G_1} or T_1	length of phase G_1
T_S, T_{G_2}, T_M	length of phases S, G_2, M
T_3 or T_{G_2M}	length of G_2+M
T_d	doubling time
I_S, I_M	S-phase index, mitotic index
LI (LI_t)	index of pulse labelling (at time t)
CL (CL_t)	index of continuous labelling (at time t)
P	number of proliferating cells
Q	number of non-proliferating cells
PF (PF_∞)	proliferative fraction (in equilibrium)
α	number of proliferating daughter cells per division
λ or λ_Q	loss rate of resting cells
λ_P	loss rate of proliferating cells
ρ	rate of exponential ("log phase") growth
Φ	cell loss factor
log	natural logarithm

List of symbols (continued)

λ_i (i=0,...) roots of the characteristic equation (6.8) in Chap. I

n   number of stages of the cell cycle in the Takahashi model

n_φ number of stages representing phase φ

a_i (i=1,...,n) passage rate in the Takahashi model

b   equal passage rate for all stages

λ_i (i=1,...,n) rate of cell loss from stage i

b_i (i=1,...,n) sum of a_i and λ_i

$d_i(t)$ (i=1,...,n) time-dependent rate of cell kill by cytotoxic agent at stage i

$z_i(t)$ (i=1,...,n) time-dependent factor of retardation caused by cytotoxic agent at stage i

REFERENCES

Aherne WA, Camplejohn RS, Wright NA (1977): An introduction to cell population kinetics. London: Edward Arnold

Amlacher E (1974): Autoradiographie in Histologie und Zytologie. Leipzig VEB Georg Thieme-Verlag

Bailey NTJ (1964): The elements of stochastic processes with application to the natural sciences. New York: Wiley

Baserga R (1981): The cell cycle. New England Journal of Medicine 304, 453-459

Bertuzzi A, Gandolfi A, Giovenco MA (1981): Mathematical models of the cell cycle with a view to tumor studies, Math. Biosci. 53, 159-188

Bhuyan BK (1977): Cell cycle related cellular lethality. In: Growth kinetics and biochemical regulation of normal and malignant cells (Drewinko and Humphrey eds.), pp. 362-375

Bhuyan BK, Fraser, Gray, Kuentzel, Neil (1973): Cell-kill kinetics of several S-phase-specific drugs. Cancer Research 33, 888-94

Bronk BV, Dienes GJ, Paskin A (1968): The stochastic theory of cell proliferation. Biophys. J. 8, 1353-98

Burnet FM (1976): Immunology, aging and cancer. San Francisco: Freeman

Camplejohn RS (1980): A critical review of the use of vincristine as a tumour cell synchronizing agent in cancer therapy. Cell Tiss. Kinet. 13, 327-335

Clarkson B (1974): Clinical applications of cell cycle kinetics. In: Handbuch der Experimentellen Pharmakologie XXXVIII/1 (Sartorelli and Johns eds.), pp.156-193

Denekamp J (1982): Cell kinetics and cancer therapy. Springfield (Illinois): Charles C. Thomas

Dibrov BF, Zhabotinsky AM, Neyfakh YuA, Orlova MP and Churikova LI (1985): Mathematical model of cancer chemotherapy. Periodic schedules of phase-specific cytotoxic agent administration increasing selectivity of therapy. Math. Biosci. 73, 1-32

Dombernowsky P and Bichel P (1976): Recycling of resting cells in the JB-2 ascites tumor after treatment with Ara-C. Cell Tiss. Kinet. 9, 9-18

Eisen M (1979): Mathematical models in cell biology and cancer chemotherapy. Lecture Notes in Biomathematics 30. Berlin Heidelberg New York: Springer

Elkind MM (1967): Sublethal X-ray damage and its repair in mammalian cells. In: Radiation Research (G. Silini ed.), pp. 558-586. Amsterdam: North Holland Publ. Comp.

Fietkau R, Friede H, Maurer-Schultze B (1984): Cell kinetic studies of the cytostatic and cytocidal effect of 1-beta-D-Arabinofuranosylcytosine on the L1210 ascites tumor, Cancer Res. 44, 1105-13

Foa P, Maiolo AT, Lombardi L, Toivonen H, Rytömaa T, Polli EE (1982): Growth pattern of the human promyelocytic leukemia cell line HL 60. Cell Tiss. Kinet. 15, 399-404

Frei E, Bickers JL, Hewlett JS, Lane M, Leary WV, Talley RW (1969): Dose schedule and antitumor studies of arabinosyl cytosine. Cancer Res. 29, 1325-32

Frobenius G (1912): Über Matrizen aus nicht negativen Elementen. Sitzungsber. Preuss. Akad. Wiss., Berlin, 456-477

Gerecke D, Hirschmann WD, Voigtmann R, Gross R (1979): Remission induction and remission maintainance in adult acute nonlymphocytic leukemia employing a modified cytostatic (COAP) regimen. Blut 39, 39-45

Gray JW (1983): Quantitative cytokinetics: cellular response to cell cycle specific agents. Pharm. Therap. 22,163-197

Gray JW and Pallavicini MG (1981): Quantitative cytokinetic analysis reviewed. In: Biomathematics and cell kinetics (M. Rotenberg ed.), pp. 107-124. Amsterdam: North-Holland/Elsevier

Grdina DJ, Meistrich ML, Meyn RE, Johnson TS, and White RA (1984): Cell synchrony techniques. I. A comparison of methods. Cell Tiss. Kinet. 17, 223-236

Guiguet M, Klein B, Valleron A-J (1978): Diurnal variation and the analysis of percent labelled mitoses curves. In: Biomathematics and Cell Kinetics (Valleron and Macdonald eds.), Amsterdam-New York-Oxford

Gunduz N (1981): Cytokinetics of tumour and endothelial cells and vascularization of lung metastases in C3H/He mice. Cell Tiss. Kinet. 14, 343-363

Hartmann NR, Gilbert CW, Jansson B, Macdonald P, Steel GG, Valleron A-J (1975): A comparison of computer methods for the analysis of fraction labelled mitoses curves. Cell Tiss. Kinet. 8, 119-124

Hadwiger H (1939): Über die Integralgleichung der Bevölkerungs-theorie. Mitteilungen d. Vereinig. schweiz. Versicherungs-mathematiker 38, 1-14

Hoppensteadt F (1975): Mathematical Theories of Populations: Demography, Genetics and Epidemics. Philadelphia: Society for Industrial and Applied Mathematics 1975

Houck JC (ed.): Chalones. Amsterdam-Oxford-New York: North-Holland/ Elsevier 1976

Jagers P (1975): Branching Processes with Biological Applications. New York: Wiley

Kellerer AM and Hug O (1972): Theory of dose-effect relations. In: Handbuch d. Med. Radiologie II/3, pp.1-42

Kendall DG (1948): On the role of variable generation time in the development of a stochastic birth process. Biometrika 35, 316-330

Keyfitz N: Introduction to the Mathematics of Population. Reading (Massachusetts): Addison-Wesley 1977

Klein B and Valleron A-J (1977): A compartmental model for the study of diurnal rhythms in cell populations. J. Theor. Biol. 64, 27-42

Klein HO and Lennartz KJ (1974): Chemotherapy after synchronization of tumor cells. Semin. Hemat. 11, 203-227

Knolle H (1983a): Kritischer Vergleich von einigen Arbeiten zum Blockierungseffekt von Cytosinarabinosid, Arzneim.-Forsch./Drug Res. 33 (II) 1507-09

Knolle H (1983b): A relation between growth fraction and cell loss factor of cell populations with distributed cycle times. Math. Biosci. 67, 167-173

Knolle H (1984a): A simple method to calculate the cell loss factor. Cell Tiss. Kinet. 17, 311-312

Knolle H (1984b): New formulae for the evaluation of a single set of data from double labelling with C14-TdR and H3-TdR. Cell Tissue Kinet. 17, 661-666

Knolle H (1986): Values of growth fraction and cell loss factor of 65 tumours reexamined, Cell Tiss. Kinet. 19, 503-509

Korr H, Schilling W-D, Schultze B, Maurer W (1983): Autoradiographic studies of glial proliferation in different areas of the brain of the 14-day-old rat. Cell Tiss. Kinet. 16, 393-413

Langen P (1980): Zellkinetik und antineoplastische Chemotherapie. In: Experimentelle und klinische Tumorchemotherapie (S. Tanneberger ed.), Vol.I, pp. 193-217. Stuttgart: Gustav Fischer

Mendelsohn ML (1975): Cell cycle kinetics and radiation therapy. In: Proceedings V. International Congress on Radiation Research (ed. O.F. Nygaard), pp.1009-24. London: Academic Press 1975

Nias AH and Fox M (1971): Synchronization of mammalian cells with respect to the mitotic cycle. Cell Tiss. Kinet. 4, 375-398

Nicolini C (1975): The discrete phases of the cell cycle: Autoradiographic, physical and chemical evidences. J. Nat. Cancer Inst. 55, 821- 826

Pallavicini MG, Gray JW, Folstad LJ (1982): Quantitative analysis of the cytokinetic response of KHT tumors in vivo to 1-beta-D-Arabinosylcytosine. Cancer Res. 42, 3125-31

Putten LM van (1974): Are cell kinetic data relevant for the design of tumor chemotherapy schedules? Cell Tiss. Kin. 7,493-504

Rubinow SI (1968): A maturity-time representation for cell populations. Biophys. J. 8, 1055-73

Rubinow SI and Lebowitz JL (1976a): A mathematical model of the acute myeloblastic state in man. Biophys. J. 16, 897-910

Rubinow SI and Lebowitz JL (1976b): A mathematical model of the chemotherapeutic treatment of acute myeloblastic leukemia. Biophys. J. 16, 1257-72

Sachs L (1986): Growth, differentiation and the reversal of malignancy. Scientific Amer. 254, 30-37

Schultze B (1969): Autoradiography at the cellular level (Physical techniques in biological research, A.W. Pollister ed., vol. III part B). New York and London : Academic Press

Schultze B, Maurer W, Hagenbusch H (1976): A two-emulsion autoradiographic technique and the discrimination of the three different types of labelling after double labelling with H3- and C14- Thymidine. Cell Tiss. Kinet. 9, 245-255

Schultze B, Kellerer AM, Maurer W (1979): Transit times through the cycle phases of jejunal crypt cells of the mouse - Analysis in terms of the mean values and the variances. Cell Tiss. Kinet. 12, 347-359

Shackney SE (1973): A cytokinetic model for heterogeneous mammalian cell populations. I. Cell growth and cell death. J. theor. Biol. 38, 305-333

Sinclair WK (1967): Radiation effects on mammalian cell populations in vitro. In: Proceedings III. Internat. Congress Radiation Research (ed. G. Silini). Amsterdam: North Holland Publ. Comp.

Skipper HE(1971): Kinetics of mammary tumor cell growth and implications for therapy. Cancer 28, 1479-99

Skipper HE and Perry S (1970): Kinetics of normal and leukemic leukocyte populations and relevance to chemotherapy. Cancer Res. 30, 1883-97

Skipper HE, Schabel FM and Wilcox WS (1964): Experimental evaluation of potential anticancer agents XIII. On the criteria and kinetics associated with curability of experimental leukaemia. Cancer Chemother. Rep. 35, 3-111

Skipper HE, Schabel FM and Wilcox WS (1965): Experimental evaluation of potential anticancer agents XIV. Further studies of certain basic concepts underlying chemotherapy of leukaemia. Cancer Chemother. Rep. 45, 5-28

Smets LA, Taminiau J, Hahlen K, de Waal F, Behrendt H (1983): Cell kinetic responses in childhood acute nonlymphocytic leukemia during high dose therapy with cytosine arabinoside. Blood 61, 79-84

Southwest Oncology Group(1974): Cytarabine for acute leukemia in adults. Arch. Int. Med. 133, 251-259

Staudte RG (1981): On the accuracy of some estimates of cell cycle time. In: Biomathematics and cell kinetics (ed. M. Rotenberg), pp. 233-242. Amsterdam: North-Holland/Elsevier

Steel GG (1968): Cell loss from experimental tumours. Cell Tiss. Kinet. 1, 193-207

Steel GG : Growth Kinetics of Tumours. Oxford: Clarendon Press 1977

Sundareshan MK and Fundakowski R (1984): On the equivalence of mathematical models for cell proliferation kinetics. Cell Tissue Kinet. 17, 609-618

Swan GW (1980): Optimal control in some cancer chemotherapy problems, Int. J. Systems Sci., vol.11, no.2, 223-237

Swan GW (1981): Optimization of Human Cancer Radiotherapy. Heidelberg: Springer

Takahashi M (1966): Theoretical basis for cell cycle analysis. I. Labelled mitosis wave method. J. Theoret. Biol. 13, 202-211

Takahashi M (1968): Theoretical basis for cell cycle analysis. II. Further studies on labelled mitosis wave method. J. Theoret. Biol. 18, 195-209

Trott KR(1972): Strahlenwirkungen auf die Vermehrung von Säuge-tierzellen. In: Handbuch Med. Radiol. II/3, p. 47

Valeriote FA and Edelstein MB (1977): The role of cell kinetics in cancer chemotherapy. Seminars in Oncology 4, 227-255

Valeriote FA and Putten L van (1975): Proliferation-dependent cytotoxicity of anticancer agents: a review. Cancer Res. 35, 2619-30

Wheeler GP, Bowdon BJ, Adamson DJ, Vail MH (1972): Comparison of the effects of several inhibitors of the synthesis of nucleic acids upon the viability and progression through the cell cycle of cultured H.Ep.No. 2 cells. Cancer Res. 32, 2661-69

Wichmann HE: Regulationsmodelle und ihre Anwendung auf die Blutbildung. Medizinische Informatik und Statistik, Nr. 48. Berlin Heidelberg New York: Springer 1984

Wielandt H (1949): Unzerlegbare, nicht negative Matrizen. Math. Zeitschrift 52, 642-648

Withers HR (1975): The four R's of radiotherapy. Adv. Radiat. Biology 5, 241-271

Wright NA, Appleton DR (1980): The metaphase arrest technique. A critical review. Cell Tiss. Kinet. 13, 643-663

Zietz S and Nicolini C (1978): Flow microfluorometry and cell kinetics. A review. In: Biomathematics and cell kinetics (ed. Valleron and Macdonald). Amsterdam-New York-Oxford 1978

SUBJECT INDEX

Abstracts, Index to Scientific Reviews, Final

Your source for advances in theoretical biology and biomathematics

Journal of Mathematical Biology

ISSN 0303-6812   Title No. 285

Editorial Board: K. P. Hadeler, Tübingen; S. A. Levin, Ithaca (Managing Editors); H. T. Banks, Providence; J. D. Cowan, Chicago; J. Gani, Santa Barbara; F. C. Hoppenstedt, East Lansing; D. Ludwig, Vancouver; J. D. Murray, Oxford; T. Nagylaki, Chicago; L. A. Segel, Rehovot

Subscription Information:
To enter your subscription, or to request sample copies, contact Springer-Verlag, Dept. ZSW, Heidelberger Platz 3, D-1000 Berlin 33, W. Germany

For mathematicians and biologists working in a wide variety of fields – genetics, demography, ecology, neurobiology, epidemiology, morphogenesis, cell biology – **the Journal of Mathematical Biology** publishes:

- papers in which mathematics is used for a better understanding of biological phenomena
- mathematical papers inspired by biological research, and
- papers which yield new experimental data bearing on mathematical models

Abstracted/Indexed in: Current Contents, Excerpta Medica, Index Medicus, Mathematical Reviews, Science Abstracts, Animal Breeding Abstracts, Compumath, Helminthological Abstracts, Index to Scientific Reviews, Plant Breeding Abstracts, Zentralblatt für Mathematik

Springer-Verlag
Berlin Heidelberg New York
London Paris Tokyo Hong Kong

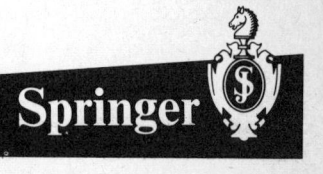

Springer

Bio-mathematics

Managing Editor: **S. A. Levin**

Editorial Board: **M. Arbib,
H. J. Bremermann, J. Cowan,
W. M. Hirsch, J. Karlin,
J. Keller, K. Krickeberg,
R. C. Lewontin, R. M. May,
J. D. Murray, A. Perelson,
T. Poggio, L. A. Segel**

Volume 15
D. L. DeAngelis, W. M. Post, C. C. Travis

Positive Feedback in Natural Systems

1986. 90 figures. XII, 290 pages. ISBN 3-540-15942-8

Contents: Introduction. – The Mathematics of Positive Feedback. –
Physical Systems. – Evolutionary Processes. – Organisms Physiology
and Behavior. – Resource Utilization by Organisms. – Social Behavior. –
Mutualistic and Competitive Systems. – Age-Structured Populations. –
Spatially Heterogeneous Systems: Islands and Patchy Regions. –
Spatially Heterogeneous Ecosystems; Pattern Formation. – Disease and
Pest Outbreaks. – The Ecosystem and Succession. – Appendices. –
References. – Subject Index. – Author Index.

Volume 16

Complexity, Language, and Life: Mathematical Approaches

Editors: **J. L. Casti, A. Karlqvist**
1986. XIII, 281 pages. ISBN 3-540-16180-5

Contents: Allowing, forbidding, but not requiring: a mathematic for
human world, – A theory of stars in complex systems. – Pictures as
complex systems. – A survey of replicator equations. – Darwinian evolu-
tion in ecosystems: a survey of some ideas and difficulties together with
some possible solutions. – On system complexity: identification, measurement, and management. – On information and complexity. –
Organs and tools; a common theory of morphogenesis. – The language
of life. – Universal principles of measurement and language functions in
evolving systems.

Volume 17

Mathematical Ecology

An Introduction
Editors: **Th. G. Hallam, S. A. Levin**
1986. 84 figures. XII, 457 pages. ISBN 3-540-13631-2

Contents: Introduction. – Physiological and Behavioral Ecology. –
Population Ecology. – Communities and Ecosystems. – Applied Mathematical Ecology. – Author Index. – Subject Index.

Volume 18

Applied Mathematical Ecology

Editors: **S. A. Levin, T. G. Hallam, L. J. Gross**
1988. ISBN 3-540-19465-7. In preparation

Volume 19
J. D. Murray

Mathematical Biology

1988. ISBN 3-540-19460-6. In preparation

Springer-Verlag
Berlin Heidelberg New York
London Paris Tokyo Hong Kong

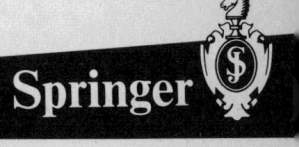